THE QUACK DOCTOR

HISTORICAL REMEDIES
FOR ALL YOUR ILLS

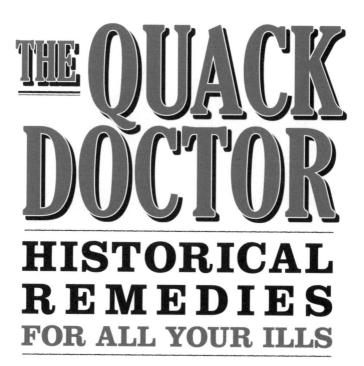

THE QUACK DOCTOR

HISTORICAL REMEDIES

FOR ALL YOUR ILLS

CAROLINE RANCE

The History Press

First published 2013

The History Press
The Mill, Brimscombe Port
Stroud, Gloucestershire, GL5 2QG
www.thehistorypress.co.uk

British Library Cataloguing in Publication Data.
A catalogue record for this book is available from the British Library.

ISBN 978 0 7524 8773 1

Typesetting and origination by The History Press
Printed in Great Britain

CONTENTS

1

A POISONOUS NOSTRUM IN ONE HAND AND THE HOLY BIBLE IN THE OTHER

The new tombstone at St Leonard's, Shoreditch, excited interest and comment. Its epitaph, cheering to the whimsical and terrifying to those with a fear of premature burial, made a change from the usual 'departed this life': Dr John Gardner, His Last and Best Bedroom, 1807.

Should you have strolled past the churchyard's boundary in 1807, you might wonder over the inscription's meaning and pause to regret the passing of the eccentric worm-doctor, privately thanking the Lord that you retained possession of life and health.

Also retaining possession of life and health, however, was Dr John Gardner, who was heartily continuing to dispense remedies at his unusual museum. Only a decline in the number of customers convinced him of the inadvisability of erecting his gravestone before he was actually dead, and tradition has it that he had the stone edited to read 'His intended Last and Best Bedroom', which must have delighted the stone mason no end.

In 1807 Gardner was 55 years old and would enjoy three more decades before taking residence in his churchyard spot. Meanwhile, he could commute on his large roan horse

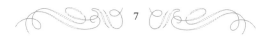

between his country estate and his shops in Long Acre and Shoreditch, make donations to religious organisations, and live well on convincing people that their every symptom was the result of one thing – *worms*.

Intestinal worms might have been more common in Gardner's time than they are in the UK today, but that doesn't mean people were blasé about them or welcomed them as pets. The 'They Were Used To It' view of history might lump worms in with hunger, cold and infant mortality as something the poor saps of t'olden days hardly noticed, but proprietary worm medicines were big business. People would do just about anything to get rid of real or suspected parasites.

Gardner's advertisements were gleeful in their fascinatingly horrible and far-fetched account of the beasts his medicine had expelled from the human body. A broadside from around 1822 describes the creatures preserved in the doctor's museum:

Worms, from 1 inch to 130 in length, some with 150 suckers; others in the form of caterpillars; another species like woodlice, 12 feet to each; a wolf of the stomach, expelled from a lady at Hoxton, who had nearly fallen victim to its ravages!!

One animal, with ears like a mouse, from a gentleman. Another with 4 horns, 6 legs, and 12 feet, which lived 9 days, from a child of 9 years; a Tape Worm, its edges like the teeth of a saw; a Stomach Worm by a lady's mouth, 7 inches long, in the act of emitting its young; male and female Teres, one emitting her young, were preying in the vitals of a gentleman five years, who could find no relief in Paris, nor Edinburgh!!!

A round Worm, 10 inches long, from the mouth of a child, aged 20 months, at the Palace; a Worm, resembling a small snake from the bowels of a man; 44 round Worms, 9 inches each, from a child; a narrow Tape Worm from a young woman's mouth, 18 feet – she also voided 40 feet downwards, had been afflicted 16 years.

An insect from a young woman's stomach, of a caterpillar form: it lived 7 weeks in a bottle, and gnawed through two corks!!

> Two hundred worms resembling wood-lice, expelled from Mr.
> A—— Hollywell Mount, which had tormented him for many
> months; a Bamboo Worm, with 4 horns and 12 legs, expelled from
> a man, whom it had nearly destroyed. Worms from the mouth, nose
> and ears of Mrs. T.——, and in the milk of the breast of Mrs. P.——,
> Bishopsgate Road.

All were bottled and displayed for the education and terror of
the potential future patient. But these specimens were not all
they appeared.

Gardner's popularity attracted attention from the anti-
quackery publications of the early nineteenth century,
including *The Medical Adviser, or, Guide to Health and Long Life*,
which printed a letter from 'An Enemy to Imposture—B',
who claimed to know the truth about the doctor's earlier life.
Gardner had served in a West India regiment, during which
time he became interested in medicine. Lack of supplies led
him to be creative with whatever was available, and when he
relieved a fellow soldier's rheumatism with a dose of gunpowder
in gin, his medical reputation was secured. 'Considering the
pill as a more dignified method than the bayonet,' said another
periodical, the *London Medical and Surgical Spectator*, 'he left off
the one, and has continued his warfare on society, we are told
very successfully, with the other.'

After leaving the army, Gardner worked for a picture framer
called Mr Floot, rising to the role of foreman and then partner
before setting up in opposition. He also became a Methodist
preacher, combining religion and medicine in a conspicuous
way that his enemies saw as hypocritical.

Gardner initially sold pills against gout, while his wife
Margaret was the proprietor of a nipple shield and ointment
for lactating mothers. They also dabbled in electrical
medicine, advertising 'The poor electrified *gratis*'. It was the
Worm Medicine, however, that would make their fortune,

and around the turn of the nineteenth century its inventor adopted the title of 'Doctor', apropos of business success rather than qualification.

Morbidly fascinating advertisements like the above-quoted handbill served to attract people to Dr Gardner's shops, but it was once they arrived that the full ghastliness of their condition became apparent. In the window, rows of bottles and jars lured the passer-by to gawp in revulsion. Within, enquirers – already concerned enough about their health to have gone there in the first place – would find themselves surrounded by an astonishing display of specimens. Suspended in preserving fluid were creatures of frightful aspect – tapeworms as thick and black as eels, reptiles with clawed hands, snail-like monsters and collections of caterpillars.

The doctor himself was likely to be 'at prayers' or in his laboratory (a closet with a sign saying 'Laboratory' above the door), so a respectable-looking and plainly dressed woman – perhaps Mrs Gardner or perhaps an employee – welcomed the patient and listened to their symptoms. She would select an exhibit from the collection and allow the patient to become acquainted with the very beast that was nibbling away inside him. The cure would cost 30*s*, but the specimens convinced enough people to do whatever it took to get their unwanted passenger out. And this is not surprising when you consider that, even if Gardner's exhibits were not all they seemed, the truth was bad enough.

The *Teres* referred to in Gardner's broadside is the round-worm species now known as *Ascaris lumbricoides*, a creature that still inhabits up to 10 per cent of the developing world's population, and is responsible for 60,000 deaths – mostly those of children – per year. The ascarid, or large roundworm, grows to about a foot long and its life cycle involves a stint in your lungs before the larvae ascend the bronchial tracts into your throat, where you would normally swallow them without noticing. If you are particularly unlucky, however, you might cough or sneeze one out. Probably onto your pillow, so that you meet him in person in the morning. An internet image search for this parasite is not recommended, but the curious will find that it brings up plenty, i.e. whatever you had for dinner, followed by whatever you had for lunch and breakfast.

The *Medical Adviser* gave the remedy's composition as saltpetre, sulphur and crude antimony, but also possible are the ingredients listed in the *London Medical and Surgical Spectator* and the *Medical Observer* – mercury, jalap, gamboge and scammony, all common components of both proprietary worm medicines and orthodox prescriptions. These 'drastic purgatives' could have spectacular effects upon the bowels, and the mercury content was dangerous, particularly where unevenly mixed medicines left high concentrations of the metal in one batch and not much in another.

It was not, however, only the physical effects of the remedies that could debilitate the patient. The worm-doctor/patient relationship could also result in psychological distress. One of Dr Gardner's clients, anonymous but for the detail that she was the wife of a coal merchant, became obsessed with the notion that a worm was wandering about her body. Originally seeking help for indigestion, she was shocked to meet face to face (or face to scolex) a preserved example of the beast afflicting her, and took Gardner's remedy for several weeks.

The medicine 'operated violently on her bowels', bringing to her chamber pot a selection of wormlike pieces, which she kept. She also suffered a probable early miscarriage, although it is impossible to know whether this would have happened anyway. Gardner assured her that his medicine would rid her of the whole creature – but if she neglected to continue the treatment, it would gnaw its way towards her heart. From then on, she began to attribute every physical discomfort to the predations of the worm. Believing the beast had lodged under her right shoulder-blade, she consulted a different doctor and was desperate enough to ask him to cut it out – a request that he politely refused.

The woman's preserved pieces of worm turned out to be undigested membranes and arteries from the meat she had eaten. Although her new physician prescribed her some medicine, he could do nothing to overcome her fear of the wandering parasite. She tried to starve it out, but the resulting hunger pains made her feel that the worm was consuming her, so she resolved to appease it by overeating, even carrying food for it in her pocket when she went out. From then on, 'her mind was so truly wretched that she seldom got any rest'.

That the woman's digestive system yielded wormlike fragments of meat highlights a fact Gardner had long been using to his advantage – lots of things look like worms.

His preserved specimens had never sojourned in the human body; they were 'the small tripe of poultry' – chicken guts suspended in such a way as to resemble tapeworms. Helpings of vermicelli played the role of smaller worms, while reptiles and insects provided further examples of supposed intestinal fauna.

Above the window display of these man-made monsters, a sign proclaimed Gardner's medicine to be 'The Universal Remedy Under God' and on the counter inside, next to the machine for electrifying the poor, sat a collecting box for the Gospel Missionaries. The incongruity between the doctor's religious activities and his apparent unconcern for the welfare of his customers inspired contempt within his critics. Portrayed as a hypocrite holding 'a poisonous nostrum in one hand and the Holy Bible in the other', he was known to harangue his patients with impromptu sermons and even attribute their failure to get better to their own lack of faith. A butcher who had suffered ill effects from the worm medicine in 1824 was surprised to discover from Gardner that working on a Sunday and not being a churchgoer had caused the trouble: 'It is an affliction of the Lord for your wickedness,' Gardner allegedly told him. 'I can do nothing for you; it would be impious to attempt relieving you. Good day – I am sorry for you, young man.'

'So am I,' replied the butcher. 'Good day, Doctor.'

But a less ostentatious side to Gardner's faith led to him founding a Christian charity that inspired philanthropy across the country and is still registered today. Back in 1785, when he had not yet achieved the fame or riches of his worm-doctoring years, Gardner established a penny-a-week subscription fund for local Methodists to contribute to the relief of the poor.

Gardner, who was not long out of the army, found himself 'called of God to visit the sick' and discovered the extent of the poverty in which many were subsisting. For all the conspicuous piety he displayed throughout his life, Gardner was perceptive enough to recognise that, 'It was to little purpose to offer comfort to the soul, when the body was the subject of gnawing hunger.' The idea of putting aside some money to help people in need came to him after he visited a miserable garret where a man was dying of a fistula. Gardner remembered:

> He lay on the floor covered with a sack, without shirt, cap, or sheet, and in a dull, despairing tone exclaimed, 'I must die without hope.' Returning home, I related to my wife these particulars and asked her if we should subscribe a penny per week each, and try to induce a few of our neighbours to do the same. In a few days the number of our infant society amounted to fifteen.

The leader of the local Methodist congregation opposed the plan, so Gardner wrote to John Wesley, who said 'I like the design and Rules of your little society' and subscribed 3d a week plus a guinea in advance. The organisation became known as the Benevolent or Stranger's Friend Society. In its first year, the Society raised £58 2s 6d, helping 1,914 people and spawning similar organisations in other British towns. Once Gardner became wealthy, he continued to give to Christian causes, donating £50 in 1823 to the British and Foreign Bible Society. All the while, he was cheerfully convincing people that snake-worms were munching away at their innards.

Gardner's attitude to his own health was possibly more circumspect. An anecdote in Bransby Cooper's biography of his uncle, Sir Astley Cooper, has the worm-doctor calling in the famous surgeon to deal with an injury. Sir Astley (at that time plain Mr Cooper) bantered with him about using his own 'Universal Remedy' but Gardner was said to have replied: 'Come, come, Dr. Cooper, *this* is a serious affair, *this* is no matter for joking!'

After a long and prosperous life, Gardner repaired at the age of 83 to his 'last and best bedroom'. The worm medicine and the displays of bottled chicken guts continued under the ownership of his grandson, John Samuel Gardner, but their heyday was over. The worms might have had a long wait, but as Gardner was lowered into the churchyard ground, they finally triumphed over their would-be nemesis.

2

WITCHCRAFT AND SUCH LIKE TOMFOOLERY

Mrs Sharp had only popped out for a bit of shopping; she never expected to come home a witch.

Something odd was certainly going on, for her neighbours had turned against her and she had been the victim of unpleasant pranks. And now the shopkeeper was giving her a meaningful look. 'Ah, that poor child is dead,' the shopkeeper said. 'Nobody can hurt it now!' On further enquiry, Mrs Sharp discovered that everyone in the neighbourhood believed she had 'overlooked' the child of one Nancy Harborough, putting the 'evil hand' upon it and cursing it to sickness and death. Drypool, Hull, had become a hotbed of witchcraft.

Yet these were not the days of the Witchfinder General, with familiars and extra nipples round every corner. It was 1844 and, as the *Hull Packet* put it, 'The facts of the case speak but little indeed for the boasted "march of intellect of the nineteenth century".'

Nancy Harborough did not invent the rumours herself – they were planted in her mind by a man calling himself Sago Jenkinson. Jenkinson enjoyed local celebrity as 'The French Doctor', in spite of being neither a doctor nor French. He was, he claimed, a Muslim from Constantinople – and this notion must have gained some credence, for the locals nicknamed him 'Dicky Mahomet'. One anonymous person, however, identified him as the son of a woman from Drypool who used to hawk greens in the streets.

Initially receiving patients at a pub and later taking his own premises, he was beseiged by people wanting his advice and was known to boast about making as much as £9 a day for dispensing medicines and wisdom. It could be difficult to get a consultation but Mrs Harborough took her child to see him at the Noah's Ark in Witham.

Perhaps unusually for a semi-itinerant practitioner, Jenkinson did not send his patient away with an expensive bottle of medicine. Instead, he (allegedly) told Mrs Harborough that her child would be cured if she did as he suggested. He informed her that she had quarrelled with a neighbour. She did not recall doing anything of the sort so he told her to come back when she remembered.

Jenkinson's temporary consulting room was so heaving with people that Mrs Harborough's next attempt to see him proved unsuccessful. But she persevered, and this time he asked her to come back in an hour with details of the supposed argument. Presumably preoccupied and frightened about her child's condition, Mrs Harborough clutched at straws and managed to dredge up a memory about the child bickering with the offspring of the unsuspecting Mrs Sharp.

His response was worthy of the inquisitors of two centuries before. Mrs Sharp had 'witched' the child, and to lift the hex, Mrs Harborough must draw blood from the witch with a pin or – better still – a worsted needle. It would be wise to make it appear an accident so as not to be arrested.

Concerned about getting in trouble with the law, Mrs Harborough abandoned the proposed assault, but did mention the doctor's strange advice to her neighbours. When her child sadly died, the gossip snowballed. The only person who didn't know about it was Mrs Sharp, minding her own business and wondering why no one seemed to like her anymore.

After her visit to the shop revealed all, Mrs Sharp, described by the local newspaper as 'a decent looking woman, about thirty-five', brought things back into the nineteenth century by instructing a lawyer. To avoid being prosecuted for slander, Mrs Harborough decided to take 'The French Doctor' to court. 'All that 'ere woman is saying is not Gospel,' the *Hull Packet* reported him as testifying, 'nor it ain't sense – except but little on it.' Amused by the case and probably keen to portray the defendant as ridiculous, the *Packet* gave a damning description of his appearance:

> The prisoner, who was exceedingly dirty in his person and linen, and who had on a grey shoddy surtout and a Prussian cap decorated with a rim of gold lace, has an emaciated appearance, and seemed when brought into court to have been indulging in spiritous liquors.

While the court did not exactly approve of Jenkinson's activities, it decided that the case was too silly to bother with. Laughter filled the courtroom when a witness for the defence called Jenkinson 'a perfect gentleman if ever there was one'.

Magistrate Mr Atkinson said it was clear Jenkinson had endeavoured to incite Mrs Harborough to a breach of the peace. He was surprised, however, to discover that anyone still believed in witchcraft these days and 'blamed the woman for her simplicity, as well as the man for his duplicity'. Atkinson hoped that the publicity of the case would stop people 'giving credence to the notions of witchcraft, and such like tomfoolery'. Sago Jenkinson was discharged and went back to his throngs of patients, who did not seem to think any the less of him.

His popularity, in fact, led to him becoming an innocent party in a case of fraud just a fortnight later. James Parsons, 30, and Thomas Trowbridge, 25, 'both of the "shabby-genteel" class', decided to cash in on the excitement surrounding the French Doctor's presence in Hull. Parsons posed as the doctor and Trowbridge, being shorter and younger, as his pupil. The two managed to convince a coughing dressmaker, Mrs Good, to buy medicine for 6s and 7d, part of which she went to borrow from a neighbour. Fortunately the neighbour had seen Jenkinson before and it became clear that the pair were imposters.

Their hearing at the Mansion House attracted a 'motley audience' who found the whole thing highly entertaining. Parsons asserted that his medicine would do as much good as any of Jenkinson's, to which the magistrate replied, 'No doubt of it.' In the opinion of a local surgeon, one bottle comprised coloured water flavoured with thyme oil, the other was 'Spanish juice [licorice], with a bitter infusion', and the pills comprised aloes and jalap – common constituents of laxatives.

Jenkinson himself appeared as a witness for the prosecution, amusing the jury and audience by revealing that 'he was not a physician; he was not a Frenchman; he had lived a great deal in France, but could not speak any French'. The prisoners were unknown to him and he had not authorised them to use his name.

At the Midsummer Quarter Sessions, Parsons and Trowbridge were acquitted on a technicality. Mrs Good had been separated from her husband for three years and did not know his whereabouts, but the likelihood was that he remained living. In the eyes of the law, therefore, the 6s and 7d were his property and Mrs Good could not bring a prosecution against Parsons and Trowbridge on her own account.

For all the laughter in court, Mrs Good still lost her money and Mrs Harborough lost her child. Tough prices to pay for a lack of education and a willingness to trust someone who might help them.

3

A SINGLE LOOK IN THE MIRROR

It is not only natural, but loveworthy in every nice woman to endeavour to look at least five years younger than she really is.

A horrid fate awaited the readers of *Myra's Journal of Dress and Fashion*. One day, they would reach the 'fatal thirty', a point of life melodramatically described as 'the knell of departed youth'. To fend off this living hell, one had to be prepared well in advance. Start lying about your age by at least 25, and the scrapheap might remain at arm's length for a few extra years.

Next to its article on the advisability of denying such wrinkledom, the *Journal* pointed interested parties in the direction of another hope of clinging to the appearance of youth – arsenic complexion wafers.

Arsenic had enjoyed a long reputation as a creator of translucent beauty and unlined skin. Its use as a cosmetic came under discussion during the sensational murder trials of Madeleine Smith in 1857 and Florence Maybrick in 1889. Both said in their defence that they had purchased arsenic for cosmetic use, Maybrick having soaked fly papers in order to extract the drug.

Maybrick's conviction for the murder of her husband revived journalistic attention to the arsenic-eaters of Styria, Austria, who had been an object of British curiosity since the middle of the nineteenth century. Sabine Baring Gould, writing in *Cassell's Magazine*, gave a description intriguing to anyone suffering the taunts of an unkind mirror:

> The arsenic eater is said to be known by the brightness, but somewhat
> metallic lustre, of the eye, by nervous excitability and irritability, by
> transparency of complexion and plumpness of flesh. Even when
> advanced in age, the arsenic-eater preserves an unusual freshness of
> appearance, and an absence of wrinkles.

But although the association between arsenic and beauty
was not new, the early 1890s saw a boom in the advertising
of commercial arsenic products specifically marketed for the
complexion. Rather than undergo the nuisance and possible
incrimination of soaking flypapers, the woman unhappy with
her looks could access a convenient and purportedly safe
beauty treatment. And far from concealing arsenic's presence,
the advertisers used it as a selling point.

Arsenic, *Myra's Journal* said, was a word to inspire terror
in those who had only heard of it as a deadly poison. They
would be surprised to discover how frequently it played a
role in medicine and how it could give a little help to the
less ethereal among us. The writer warned readers not to
take arsenic preparations without medical advice, but her
opinion was clear – 'when the nerves are good and the
complexion not all it might be, a decided improvement in
the latter might follow a course of the small Homoeopathic
Complexion Wafers prepared by Mr S Harvey, 12, Gaskarth
Road, Balham'.

The journal also accepted advertisements for the product
and recommended it on the 'agony' pages to correspondents
seeking a transformation in their problematic skin.

The wafers (i.e. tablets) and their accompanying arsenical
soap were not advertised as homoeopathic, but the term's use
in *Myra's Journal* suggests that they were known as such, and
it is likely that they followed the example of the American
products that inspired them by containing minuscule quantities
of the poison.

Their brand name was Dr MacKenzie's Harmless Arsenic Complexion Wafers, and they were probably less dangerous than their proprietor – an elusive and rather unsavoury person named Sidney J. Hawke. By the time he began selling the pills, Hawke was the wrong side of that fatal 30 but, not being a woman, he was sufficiently presentable to earn the description 'a fashionably dressed young man' during a court appearance in 1892.

His trouble with the law, however, was not for selling poison. Hawke suspected that his wife Catherine, to whom he had been married for only six months, had remained in contact with a former lover, William Dusildorff. She had previously had a baby with Dusildorff and lived 'under his protection' until immediately before her marriage, afterwards continuing to correspond with and meet Dusildorff for news of the child. Hawke tried to put a stop to this by sending a menacing postcard to Dusildorff's business address:

> Even your correspondence and telegrams are in safe keeping. At your every meeting you will be followed and watched. You shall bitterly repent it. I am not to be trifled with. It is owing to you and another that I am separated from my wife and my home broken up. The other has paid the penalty, and will show it to his dying day. Your turn is to come in due course. Very well, you shall pay for it.

On this occasion the judge ordered that he enter into his own recognisances of £500 to keep the peace for twelve months. Later that year Mr and Mrs Hawke, plus dog, set sail for the U.S., returning to London in June 1893.

Within a fortnight, advertisements for 'Dr Campbell's Harmless Arsenic Complexion Wafers' appeared in the London papers, promising to 'produce the most Lovely Complexion that the imagination could desire, no matter what condition it may be in now'.

Dr Campbell's New York-based brand (which used 'safe' rather than 'harmless' in its name) had been around since about 1887 and its proprietor claimed to have made the wonderful discovery when despairing about his own sallow face. Until the age of 19 he 'was the possessor of a remarkably clear skin and bright English complexion, so much so as to excite comment among my fellow college students, who used to say "they wished I were a girl"'.

Yellow fever, however, put the kybosh on his friends' adoring glances, and rendered Dr Campbell 'a far deeper yellow than Oscar Wilde's favourite sunflower'. Only his own arsenic formulation managed to restore him to general admiration. And of course, it could do the same for the purchaser.

Back in London, Hawke's company, S. Harvey, advertised as the sole UK agent for the Campbell wafers, but it is difficult to ascertain whether this was official or whether Hawke simply recognised a niche in the British market and sought to fill it by ripping off Campbell's adverts. The brand soon disappeared, to be replaced by Dr MacKenzie's Harmless Arsenic Complexion

ONE BOX OF DR. MACKENZIE'S IMPROVED HARMLESS ARSENIC WAFERS

will produce the most lovely complexion that the imagination could desire ; clear, fresh, free from blotch, blemish, coarseness, redness, freckles, or pimples. Sent post free for 4s 6d. —S. HARVEY (Dept. 32), 12, Gaskarth Road, Balham Hill, London, S.W. To whiten hands and skin use Dr. Mackenzie's Arsenical Toilet Soap, 1s. 3d. per tablet, post free, three for 1s. 9d.

Arsenic Wafers. *Author's collection*

Wafers, but the advertising details remained the same, from the phrasing of the copy to the picture of a young woman whispering her beauty secret to a friend.

Just as the brand was getting established, Hawke's presence graced the police courts again after he was violent to Catherine, seizing her by the throat and, when she escaped and ran out of the house, locking her out in the rain until seven o'clock the next morning. Although he denied that the attack took place and claimed that Catherine had threatened to shoot him, the magistrate deemed him guilty of a 'cowardly assault' and fined him £5. Catherine was granted a divorce in 1897 after detailing his cruelty and adultery throughout their marriage.

Dr MacKenzie's Arsenical Toilet Soap appeared in 1895, with a sneaky introduction to the market via the newspapers' personal ads:

> Dearest Cora – Have you noticed how much Georgie's complexion has improved lately? He has been using Dr MacKenzie's arsenical toilet soap. Have you tried it? It is simply delicious. Yours with fondest love Martha.

The soap, a delightfully perfumed, good quality product, proved immediately popular and when shares in S. Harvey (Limited) were released for subscription in 1897, the prospectus stated that sales had reached 340,000 pieces a year.

And yet there were no reports of people dropping dead as a result of using the soap and its many imitators. Could they be as harmless as the adverts claimed?

During 1896 and 1897, several chemists received court summons under the Sale of Food and Drugs Act for selling arsenical soap, whether they had made it themselves or bought it in good faith from a supplier. And yet, the offence was not that it contained arsenic – it was that it *didn't* contain arsenic.

Analysis of samples collected by secret shoppers showed that arsenical soaps contained either negligible quantities of the metal or none whatsoever, and the product could not therefore be considered 'of the nature, substance, and quality' demanded by the purchaser. In their defence, the chemists claimed that the soap simply had a 'fancy name' intended to appeal to the prevailing interest in arsenic as a beauty aid.

One chemist, Septimus Walgate of Ealing, used one-sixth of a grain (10.8mg) of arsenic per hundredweight of soap. None was discernible in the sample bar and Walgate's comment that Sunlight Soap didn't contain any sunlight either was not enough to get him out of being fined.

In response to these cases, S Harvey Ltd recalled chemists' stocks of Dr MacKenzie's soap and replaced them with a new formula, reassuring their retailers that it now had more arsenic and indemnifying them against prosecution. 'Possibly now,' said *The Lancet*, 'if the soap is used indiscriminately by the public there will be some cases of arsenical poisoning. That, however, is for the public to guard against.'

An anonymous West End chemist interviewed by *Hearth and Home* in 1897 referred to the proliferation of adverts and the implied popularity of their products as 'the Arsenic Craze'. But if such a craze existed, then part of it was among writers taking the opportunity to propagate a morality tale on the dangers of female vanity.

The image of the other-worldly beauty, her alabaster skin disguising the deadly poison at work inside her, was worthy of a fairy tale in which the heroine's vanity leads her to sell her life for temporary beauty. Stories of arsenic use in Australia told of a woman captivating a man with her beauty and then revealing after marriage that the poison had made her bald. And once within arsenic's grasp, the victim was trapped, her only choices being to continue taking the poison until it killed her, or to give it up and see her looks wither to a worse state than she could ever have imagined:

> Even a few weeks' abandonment of the drug will convert her languorous beauty into faded ugliness. The skin assumes the tint of ancient whitewash. The nose grows flabby, and the hue which so adorns the cheek capriciously establishes itself at the tip of that olfactory organ. The head grows heavy, and the nervous system, like the heroine of any paper covered romance, is torn with contending emotions. A single look in the mirror makes this wretched creature an arsenic consumer once more.

Fortunately for the consumer of commercial arsenic products like MacKenzie's wafers and soap, such a fate was averted. Those desperate to transform an unsatisfactory complexion were better – or worse – off sticking to the fly papers.

4

EVERY AFFECTION INCIDENTAL
TO THE HUMAN FRAME

On 19 January 1838, the steamer *Killarney* set sail from Cork, bound for Bristol. On board were thirty-seven people and 600 pigs, and ahead of them was the most violent storm in more than half a century. The steamer was forced to turn back and anchored at Cove for a few hours until her captain made the ill-fated decision to continue. By the following evening, twenty-one survivors were clinging to a rock, fast losing hope of rescue.

One of these survivors was Baron Spolasco, a flamboyant character who had been practising as a physician and surgeon in different parts of Ireland. Yet as he confronted a watery death within sight of land on that January night, his adventures had only just begun.

Although Spolasco's name and portrait appear exotic, he started life as John Smith in the north of England in the first decade of the nineteenth century. The exact date of his birth is difficult to trace, as he seems to have approached middle age with some reluctance, knocking a few years off when the opportunity arose. But whatever his origins, his career was characterised by fame, fortune, shipwreck, prison, Byronic melodrama, ruffled shirts, gold spectacles and various illegitimate children. For as well as claiming for his medical abilities: 'the Consumptive cured – the Cripple made to walk

– the Deaf to hear – the Dying to live – the Blind to see, and every other affection treated incidental to the human frame', Spolasco was, to be frank, a bit of a shagger.

He had his own range of patent medicines, including the 'Life Preservers' – an anti-biliousness remedy – the 'Wash of Syria' for beautifying the skin and 'The Poor's Treasure, or the Green Healing Ointment of Venice', for hives. His advertisements also imply that he could advise ladies on contraception, though he does not seem to have extended this service to his own servant girls. He did not, however, confine his talents to medicine – he could turn his delicate white hand to surgery too. A brief but interesting section of his handbills read: 'Any individual who has lost his, or her nose, can be supplied with a REAL one, Grecian, Roman or Aquiline, perfect and natural as by nature.' This referred to the Talicotian operation, an ancient and ingenious way of reconstructing a missing nose (often a consequence of syphilis) by bringing down a flap of skin from the patient's forehead. Spolasco's later pamphlets trumpet the case of Patrick Sheahan from County Clare, who was noseless for twenty years. The Baron carried out the operation and, 'notwithstanding he bled profusely', Sheahan emerged as the possessor of a perfect Roman example.

On that fateful Friday in January 1838, however, Spolasco was off to Bristol to meet the agent of a 'high personage' about a complicated surgical case. At least that was what he later told his public; it's also possible that the residents of Cork were getting wise to (or *enceinte* by) him and he felt it prudent to leave. All his belongings were loaded onto the *Killarney* but he, his 8-year-old son Robert and their two Newfoundland dogs were five minutes late. They had almost resolved to wait for the next week's boat, when some locals offered to row them out to the steamer.

During the course of that night and the next morning the storm terrified the pigs, who all crowded to one side, putting the steamer in peril and at last causing it to perish in Renny Bay. The poor Newfoundlands rapidly joined the choir invisible, but the Baron and Robert were among the twenty-one people who reached a rock 200 yards from shore. Though so close to land, there were no rescue attempts until the Sunday, by which time little Robert was among those who had succumbed to the waves. In his *Narrative of the Wreck of the Steamer Killarney*, Spolasco later described his feelings about the death of his son:

> I pause one moment to offer up my most fervent supplications to my God, to spare such of you my kind readers, as are fathers, and mothers; to spare you ever, from having to go through, to witness, to feel, to suffer, even a thousandth part of what I did for my dear, my sweet, my beautiful boy. Alas! he is now no more, he is as still as the grave! yes

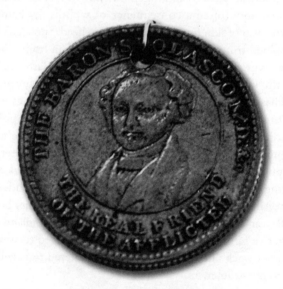

Baron Spolasco advertising token.
Courtesy of Lucy Martin, www.roundography.com

he is quiet – he moves not – he breathes not – he no longer enchants me as he was wont to do, morning, noon and night, with his sweet prattling, his but too sensible conversation! HE IS DEAD!!!

The *Narrative* is a gripping read and, while saturated with melodrama, concurs in most details with other reports of the wreck.

We had not the good fortune to reach the top of the rock; we only got to between one and two yards of it and that part faced the sea. We had to hold on all night by our fingers and toes – something like being suspended by our hands and toes from the sill of a window in one of the upper stories of a house, and at every moment the tremendous and fearful billows lashing at our backs terribly, we were not able to rest ourselves even for a moment.

The drama is heightened by just how close the stranded people were to the shore. During the hours of daylight, they could see the locals making off with the dead pigs washed up on the beach, but the treacherous waves crashed between them and safety.

Eventually they were spotted by some 'respectable' people who sent for a set of rescue apparatus, but this relied on conveying a rope the 200 yards to the rock and attempts proved futile. The rescuers tried attaching ropes to ducks and setting them off across the waves, but only one duck made it and refused to be caught by the survivors. Next they tried using a howitzer to fire balls with ropes attached, but to no avail.

Then the chief coastguard's brother, Edward Hull, had the idea of carrying a long rope all the way around the bay so that it would stretch from one cliff to the other, with a second rope hanging down over the rock. The first attempt was late on Sunday afternoon and as darkness fell the rescuers almost left off, but in desperation two people grabbed the rope and shouted to be hauled in. According to the Baron, '[the rescuers] immediately did so, upon which we heard a splash but could see nothing, it being at this time dark'.

After this melancholy occurrence, the remaining survivors were abandoned to a second night without food, water or shelter. The next day, using the long rope and a basket, those on land were finally able to get the staples of life – wine, whisky and bread – onto the rock. The Baron wrote:

> I cannot find words sufficiently strong to express how grateful the wine was to my parched lips. Each having partaken of this seasonable relief, we all huzza'd, and waved our hats and caps, in token of gratitude for what we had just had, and in the hope of being speedily relieved.

The equipment included a cot designed to transport human beings and by this method the fourteen survivors were removed, one by one. First was the only woman, Mary Leary, but Baron Spolasco made sure he was second in line and was taken to a nearby house. One of the others subsequently died of exhaustion.

Only a month later he wrote his *Narrative* and used it as a way of increasing his fame and spreading the word about his medical practice. He went through with his plan of going to Bristol, arriving there with the claim that he had just returned from a tour through the principal cities of Europe. He gave patients an impression of his popularity by advertising how difficult it was to get to see him:

> In consequence of the number of sufferers who daily crowd round Baron Spolasco's consulting rooms, he has found it necessary, in order to save his valuable time, to charge an admission fee of 5s., which admission fee, if the patient be poor, will be received as consideration for the Baron's advice; the wealthy will, of course, have to pay the usual fee of a guinea.

Baron Spolasco next moved on to Swansea and celebrated the first anniversary of his rescue by paying for a whole ox to be distributed among the poor. He was, however, about to suffer a temporary reversal of his fortunes. Just a few weeks later, he was arrested and charged with the manslaughter of a young woman.

Twenty-two-year-old Susannah Thomas had visited Spolasco about abdominal pain. The evidence given by her aunt, Elizabeth Arnott, at the inquest gives an insight into how he worked. The Baron allegedly:

> told [Miss Thomas] he knew by her eyes, that she was very ill, and that he would cure her; afterwards she would have cause to bless the hour she saw the good Baron Spolasco. Witness was not allowed to relate the symptoms of the disorder of deceased to the Baron, as he said he could know them by her bold eye.

In return for 22s 6d, he supplied two pills folded in pink-and-blue paper and some powder folded in white paper – Mrs Arnott noticed that this was exactly the same for all the other patients, regardless of what was wrong with them. Back home, Miss Thomas became worse, so her aunt sent for the Baron, who advised her to try some castor oil and a gruel and turpentine enema. A quarter of an hour after he left, Miss Thomas died. The autopsy revealed that her intestines were inflamed and her stomach ulcerated and gangrenous, with a hole in the stomach wall allowing the contents to escape into her abdominal cavity. The surgeon conducting the post mortem examination believed that the Baron's medicines – composed of aloes and jalap – had hastened the patient's death.

Baron Spolasco, furious about the 'foul conspiracy got up against him' was sent to Cardiff gaol to await the next County Sessions. Having the cash to stump up bail, however, he immediately got out. When his trial came up, the surgeon

Most important to all classes of Society!!

Just arrived from the Continent, the singularly gifted, highly talented and

Celebrated Doctor Baron SPOLASCO, M. D.

And M.R.C.S. K.O.M.T. & C.L. D'H.

The most successful Practitioner of the two Professions, both surgery and Medicine, of any other in the known World,

Will have the honor of visiting ~~~~ 1837, and may be personally consulted, by each sex, for a short time, daily, at his Residence, ~~~~ on all cases, both Medical and Surgical, that human nature is heir to, between the hours of Ten in the morning, and Four in the afternoon; and in the evening from Six till Nine.

The Baron is a Licentiate Physician, and Member of the Royal College of Surgeons, and was a perpetual Pupil to the late celebrated Baron Dupuytren, of the Hotel Dieu, Paris, having studied the various branches of the Two Professions, at the Universities and Colleges of London, Edinburg, Dublin, Glasgow, Paris, and other Schools on the Continent. Diplomas and certificates of qualification, and certificates of cures, can be seen.

Those *Married Ladies,* whose *Child-birth* is to them *almost death itself,* need never again be in *that way,* by making timely application to the celebrated Baron.

The Baron is a First-rate Scientific Surgical Operator, and Bone-setter, and the most successful Practitioner in the treatment of Sprains and Dislocated Joints, of all others in the known world—quite alone he stands in this, his practice, which is peculiar only to himself.

Any individual who has lost his, or her nose, can be supplied with a REAL one, Grecian, Roman, or Aquiline, perfect and natural as by Nature; also the Consumptive cured, —the Cripple made to walk—the Deaf to hear—the Dying to live—the Blind to see, and every other affection treated incidental to the human frame—the Jaundice, Inflammations, Indigestions, Billous or Nervous affections, Gout, Rheumatism, Green Sickness, Cholera Morbus, Ague, Apoplexy, St. Vitus's Dance, Colds, Coughs, Gravel, Costiveness, Worms, Small Pox, Eruptions of the Skin, Want of Appetite, Dry Skin, Sickness, Flatulency, Eructations, Palpitation of the Heart, Pains of the Head and Stomach, Nausea, Frightful Dreams, Diarrhœa, Depraved Vision, Scrofula, Blotches, and all diseases of the Skin, Diabetes, Seminal Weakness, Scald Heads, Measles, Lumbago, Leprosy, Sore Eyes, Abscesses, Asthma, periodical, constitutional and spasmodic, Ulcerated Breasts, Piles, Pleurisy, Erisipelas, Croup in children, Convulsions, Cholic, Burns and Bruises, Bowel Complaints, Heartburn, Quinzy, Itch, Influenza, Dropsy, in all its stages, Contraction of the Limbs, Cancers and White Swellings, Cramp in the Stomach, Liver Complaints, Putrid Sore Throats, Impotency, Hysterics, Gleet, Fistula, Epilepsy, Paralytic, Stone and Gravel, without cutting, Swellings in the Neck, Strictures, Hectic, Spitting of Blood, Difficulty of Urine, Fits, Dysentery, Diseases created by the injudicious use of Mercury, Ruptures, Scurvy, Syphilis, or the Venereal Disease, Gonorrhœa, Corns completely eradicated, Insanity successfully treated, &c. &c. &c.

Lameness, caused by the contraction of the sinews of the knee, can be effectually cured by the Baron, although of forty years duration; and those who use crutches or stilts, be enabled to walk well without them.—On the correctness of this, the Doctor hazards his valuable professional reputation. All persons so affected will do well to make immediate application—he having performed thousands of Miraculous Cures, which were previously pronounced, by his Medical and Surgical Brethren, to be Incurable; in consequence of which the Baron stands unrivalled in his profession. He refers to his Pamphlet for a history of extraordinary cases by him treated and cured; and his invaluable Patent Medicines, viz. "The Ladies companion to the Toilet, or the wash of Syria, or beautifyer of the skin," removing all freckles, blotches and discolourations, leaving it clear and white. —" The Cordial Balm of Spolasco," for the enfeebled and debilitated of both sexes, affording them, in every relaxation, no matter from what cause, muscular strength, the desired energy, and heartfelt felicity.—"The Life Preservers, or Incomparable Vegetable anti-Bilious Family Pills;" night and morning boxes.—"The Vegetable Female, or anti-Scorbutic Drops," for the irregularities of Females, Scrofula, Scurvy, Strictures, Cancerous and fungus sores, and all eruptions of the skin.—"The Diuretic, or anti-Dropsical Pills," for the Dropsical, and for scarcity of urine—"The Poor's Treasure, or the Green Healing Ointment of Venice," for the White Hives, and all malignant ulcers and sores.—"The enamelled Tooth Powder or Fragrant Dentifrice."—Teeth and Stumps extracted on a new but unerring principle. Midwifery practised—Barrenness of Females, and all the defects peculiar to their sex, removed.

The Doctor pledges himself not to undertake any case, either in Surgery or Medicine, but what he will cure.—A certain Disorder quickly cured.—*Advice to the Poor, Gratis.*

Baron Spolasco Handbill, 1837.
Courtesy of Lucy Martin, www.roundography.com

could not say with certainty that the medicines were the cause of death so he was found not guilty.

But it wasn't long before he had another brush with the law. In March 1840 he was arrested for forging the government stamps on his pills. An undercover policeman went to the Baron's house and was furnished with medicines whose stamps imitated a design discontinued in 1823. Spolasco's defence was that the packets were intended for sale in Ireland, where stamps were not necessary. He was again sent to the Assizes and acquitted.

One might have expected him to lie low for a while after this troublesome time, but he was as ostentatious as ever and within a few months of getting out of gaol, he published a song (in both English and Welsh) lauding his genius.

> I pledge unto Spolasco's name,
> A name in which we glory;
> His splendid cures and healing fame
> Recorded are in story.
> Be mindful of Spolasco's skill,
> Ye patrons of his merit;
> Save him from all impending ill.
> And a relentless spirit.

It goes on in the same vein for ten verses.

The Baron remained in Swansea for several more years and was mentioned in an inquest for the Reverend Edward Matthews Davies, who died of kidney disease in 1843. Spolasco was accused of trying to get him to hand over 20 guineas for a consultation. Mr Davies's servant asked whether such a large amount of money would actually result in a cure and Baron Spolasco allegedly replied: 'Do you think I would take any man's money if I could not cure him? It is not the money I want, it is a name; I can get money as fast as I can count it.'

It proved clear that the Reverend Mr Davies had died of natural causes and this time the Baron was not charged with anything. The coroner observed that:

> however culpable it might be to extort money from the pockets of a person labouring under a deadly disease, by pretending to cure him, yet a coroner's jury could not deal with the case, unless it were proved that death was caused by the medicine prescribed.

Spolasco subsequently moved to Badgeworth, near Cheltenham, receiving patients at 'Spolasco's Villa' there on Mondays and Tuesdays, at the Crown Hotel in Worcester on Wednesdays, in Birmingham every Thursday and Friday and at Swindon for three days at the beginning of each month. In spite of this demanding schedule, he found time to impregnate one of his servants, Hannah Dawe, who in February 1848 'bore in her arms a little pledge of affection' as she appealed to the Gloucester city magistrates to force Spolasco to take responsibility. The court ordered him to pay her 5s a week for the first six weeks of the baby's life, 2s 6d a week thereafter, plus 10s for the midwife.

Spolasco did not attend court in person, however. By this point he was long gone to London (where he'd spent some time already, judging by the birth of little John Spolasco to one Hannah Watkins of Enfield in July 1847). The Baron started out in lodgings before taking premises opposite the Surrey Theatre on Blackfriars Road and printing pamphlets announcing his arrival.

More attention from the courts was to come, however. A patient 'whose face was in a dreadful state from extensive cancer' complained that he had paid over £7 for medicines that made his condition worse. He got his money back but Spolasco was soon in trouble again.

A 16-year-old servant, Caroline Hearne, was accused of stealing a diamond ring from him, saying in her defence that she had taken it in revenge after he criminally assaulted her. She subsequently changed her story to state that he had 'taken a little liberty' but that she had pushed him away. Whatever the truth, the Baron denied her allegations, indignantly claiming that: 'It was not likely that a person in his condition of life would so disgrace himself as to be on intimate terms with so young a female.'

Mr Cottingham, the magistrate, dryly stated that he 'could say nothing about that'.

London evidently wasn't proving as fertile a ground for Spolasco as the provinces. A few months later, undaunted by his previous experience with boats, he boarded the ship *Wisconsin* as a cabin passenger to New York. With him was another of his illegitimate children, 7-year-old Julia. They took rooms on Broadway and Spolasco immediately set about proclaiming his miracles and charging hefty fees for his medical expertise. Within a few years, Julia had a little half-brother, William,* but their sire was rapidly going to seed. Walt Whitman's description of him in 'Street Yarn' (1856) was merciless:

> Somebody in an open barouche, driving daintily. He looks like a doll; is it alive? We'll cross the street and so get close to him. Did you see? Fantastic hat, turned clear over in the rim above the ears; blue coat and shiny brass buttons; patent leathers; shirt-frill; gold specs; bright red cheeks, and singularly definite jetty black eyebrows, moustache, and

---

* William Spolasco (b. 1853) became a policeman, as did his own son, William Augustus. The latter, 'a Hercules in size and strength', was charged with extortion in 1900, accused of attempting to secure $2,000 from Mrs Elizabeth Fitzgerald, a.k.a. Madame Zingari the Palmist Queen, to arrange her release from prison. He was acquitted.

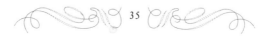

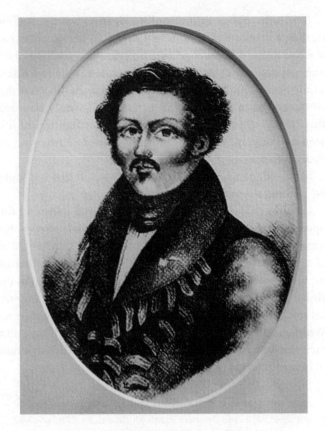

Baron Spolasco Portrait. *Author's collection*

imperial. You could see that from the sidewalk; but you saw, when you stood at his wheel, not only the twinkling diamond ring and breast-pin, but the heavy, slabby red paint; and even the substratum of grizzly gray under that jetty dye; and upon our word there's a hair of the same straggling out under the jaunty oiled wig! How straight he sits, and how he simpers, and how he fingers the reins with a delicate white little finger stuck out, as if a mere touch were all – as if his whole hand might govern a team of elephants! The Baron Spolasco, with no end

young man was troubled. Local surgeon Mr J.J. Ely said of the pamphlets: 'I have no doubt whatever they would cause a great depression of spirits.'

A leading authority on the subject, William Acton, described spermatorrhoea not just as the loss of semen but as a resulting state of enervation characterised by general debility, insomnia, 'nervous affections' and indigestion. He recognised that the term was vague enough to encompass more or less any symptom and unprincipled practitioners were quick to use this to their advantage.

In Acton's view, the major causes of the condition were masturbation and venereal excess – intercourse more than once every seven to ten days was potentially debilitating for a healthy married man. Disreputable patent remedy vendors latched onto these causes – by overplaying the dire consequences of vice, they could defraud victims of large sums of money and rely on them being too embarrassed to tell anyone.

De Roos's pamphlets were far from unique. Another notorious practitioner, Dr Henery, the pseudonym of John Osterfield Wray, used his *Vital Hints on Health and Strength* to instil fear and shame into his readers. Of the young men who had consulted him in a state of mental and physical infirmity, he said:

> I have found it a work of much time and difficulty to effect a complete cure – to snatch them from death – from the early graves to which they were hastening. Some of these were afflicted with distressing wasting dreams, nervousness, unfitness for study or business, trembling, dizziness, restlessness, palpitation of the heart, pains in the loins, and a constant sense of weariness, starting during sleep, failure of memory, frequent headache, dimness of sight, indifference to life, its hopes and pleasures, fear of insanity, and silent wretchedness from fear of impotence. The symptoms in almost all cases are from the ghastly curse – the fatal habit of self-abuse.

[Entered at Stationer's Hall.]

Ponder well before you destroy this. Small as it appears, the matter is well worth "inwardly digesting."

VITAL HINTS

ON

HEALTH AND STRENGTH;

AND THEIR DEPENDENCE ON THE STATE OF THE GENERATIVE ORGANIZATION;

WITH NOTICES ON

FUNCTIONAL DEBILITY, SPERMATORRHŒA;

AND ON THE

Curative Efficacy of Galbanic Electricity.

BY

DR. HENERY,

Author of "Human Physiology; or, The Golden Key to Health," &c., &c.,

53, DORSET STREET, MANCHESTER SQUARE, LONDON.

Read not to contradict—weigh and consider.

VITAL HINTS.

In the publication of the following observations my object is to diminish, and, if I can, to suppress, some of the most deplorable and fatal evils—moral, social, and physical—that have ever preyed upon society.

Morbid affections of the Generative Organs have been productive of a greater amount of misery, degradation, despair, disease, and premature death, than the total of all the other maladies which afflict human beings. Indeed, many affections which are sometimes treated as distinct local or constitutional disorders, are only the results and symptoms of neglected, and perhaps unsuspected, derangement of those delicate organs. The result of my own experience, and of conferences with many men eminent for medical and scientific skill, is, that a large number of the diseases that pass under various designations are merely complications or results,

Dr Henery – Vital Hints. *Image © Bodleian Library, University of Oxford 2008: John Johnson Collection, Patent Medicines 15 (41). Copyright © 2008 ProQuest LLC. All rights reserved*

Dr Henery's skill with galvanic electricity, together with his Life-Preserving Drops, would rescue the reader from the consequences of his own vice.

One of the 'Detector' letters (which Courtenay collected into a book called *Revelations of Quacks and Quackery* in 1865) cites the case of an anxious young man who responded to an advertisement placed by Dr Hammond, inventor of the 'Electric, Curative and Phosphoric Vitalizer'. The reply asked for two guineas for a 'self-curative' belt – the man sent the money but the package he received contained only 'some bottles of medicine and a lotion to rub over the penis and testicles'. Annoyed that he didn't get the belt, the patient wrote back, asking where it was.

Hammond responded with a missive calculated to scare his patient half to death. He had looked further into the case (even though he had never actually seen the man) and decided 'a slight disease of the kidneys' was causing semen to drain away.

> This vital waste is not only capable of causing all the symptoms you detail, but such is the sympathy existing between the generative functions and the brain, that should this drain of the most vital of all your secretions be not immediately arrested, your whole system must suffer very serious derangement, whilst the organs of generation themselves will become vitiated and relapse into a state of utter impotency.

This would result in complete loss of erectile function and lead to 'withering and wasting of the penis'. In case the lad wasn't already terrified enough, Hammond predicted that his case would end in insanity. Fortunately, he had sought help just in time.

Hammond again recommended the curative belt (which the patient thought he'd already paid for) and sent a bill for a further 2 guineas. The young man paid up and while it would be easy to ridicule him for throwing good money after bad, there's no law against being inexperienced and scared that there's something seriously wrong with you.

The belt arrived and proved to be an ordinary suspensory bandage with a band that went round the patient's waist, holding up a circular string of metal pieces through which one had to place the penis. This would somehow provide 'a continuous current of electricity, which is taken up by the whole system, infusing new life and "manly vigour" into the debilitated or relaxed frame, and affords great support and comfort to the testicles and generative organs'. The patient subsequently consulted Courtenay and was reassured that there was nothing wrong with him.

As well as the belts, Hammond sold Restorative Powders and Seminal Replenisher, which were not only supposed to produce top-quality semen, but also restore 'brain fluid'. In 1869, the more famous electric belt manufacturer, the Pulvermacher Company, tried to gain an injunction against Hammond for using the trademarked slogan 'Electricity is Life' – and for bringing the whole electric belt business into disrepute – but failed as it proved difficult to find out exactly who Hammond was.

Placed adjacent to Hammond's advertisements were those for what appeared to be competing specialists in electrical medicine. H. James, Medical Electrician to the London Hospitals, was promoting a belt to:

> Sufferers from Nervous Debility, Painful Dreams, Mental and Physical Depression, Palpitation of the Heart, Noises in the Head and Ears, Indecision, Impaired Sight and Memory, Indigestion, Prostration, Lassitude, Depression of Spirits, Loss of Energy and Appetite, Pains in the Back and Limbs, Timidity, Self-Distrust, Dizziness, Love of Solitude, Groundless Fears, &c.

James's address – Percy House, Bedford Square, London – and Hammond's premises at 11 Charlotte Street were, however, the same place and Henry James was either a sidekick of Hammond's or possibly even the same person. Further aliases joined the team – Dr Walter Jenner, Dr Harrison, Mr Raphey and Mr A. Barrows, all at slightly different versions of the same address. People enquiring by post from all over the country would have no reason to know this. Once patients gave up on the useless treatment from one alias, they would receive a pamphlet extolling the superior virtues of another.

Hammond also employed what Courtenay referred to as 'the hospital dodge'. His earlier ads proclaimed him to be 'of the Lock Hospital' and his letterhead described him as 'F.A.S., F.S.A., M.R.A.S., H.G. St Mary's, King's College, The Lock and St George's Hospitals, LONDON.' An impressive list – but F.A.S., F.S.A. and M.R.A.S. didn't stand for any recognised qualifications and H.G. simply meant 'Honorary Governor'.

Any Tom, Dick or Harry could become an honorary governor just by making a charitable subscription to the hospital. Although the Lock cancelled Hammond's donations when they found out what he was up to, this didn't stop him continuing to deceive patients by claiming affiliation with these respectable institutions.

Courtenay identified an interesting connection between Hammond's practice and that of Dr Henery, who was sentenced to two years' imprisonment in 1864 when a patient had the gumption to have him charged with conspiracy to defraud. The person calling himself H. James had received the same patient at Dr Henery's and Dr Hammond's premises at different times. His real identity remains uncertain but his activities hint at strong links between these businesses.

Dr Alfred Field Henery, a.k.a. John Osterfield Wray, was brought to justice by a young army captain called Montague Clarke, who braved being called 'silly' by the *British Medical*

Journal to expose Henery's attempt to blackmail him. A common sales method employed by those of Henery's ilk was to send unsolicited books and pamphlets to soldiers. Clarke either saw an advert or received one of these publications at his barracks and, the next time he was in London, called on Dr Henery for advice about spermatorrhoea. The advice was minimal but Clarke paid 11 guineas for it plus a supply of medicine, which he reordered several times, spending a total of £85.

Wray, 28, was the son of former ship's surgeon and chemist, Martin Osterfield Wray, who sold his own range of patent remedies. These included Balsamic Pills for gonorrhoea, Specific Drops for seasickness, Essence of Jamaica Ginger for cholera, an influenza mixture and Wray's Licensed Victuallers Digestive, Dinner and Liver Pills for gently opening the bowels. In spite of this heritage, however, family relations were strained. In 1860, John was arrested for putting his father in fear of bodily injury. He was not the type to have any qualms about threatening people.

So it was that, some months after Montague Clarke had received proper medical advice and given up on Dr Henery, he received a visit from Wray's alcoholic accomplice, William Anderson, with a demand for £150. When Clarke refused to pay, Anderson reduced the sum, eventually managing to get a sovereign out of him for a taxi and departing. Wray and his sidekick, however, did not give up.

They threatened to inform Clarke's employers and family that he had been treated for 'spermatorrhoea, brought on by self-pollution'. (Clarke himself maintained that his condition was due to having been shot in the head during the Crimean War.) Refused further access to the captain's accommodation, Anderson wrote to him saying:

> Now, supposing I was to inform you application would be made at the War Office, with an explanation of case, and if we were to do

so you know what the consequence would be; or supposing I was to inform you I expected to be in your neighbourhood in Scotland next week, and that I do not intend leaving here, in the event of your still persisting in your refusal to pay, without making known in the neighbourhood for what purpose I am here. I am in no hurry, and will allow you time to reflect whether it will be better to pay Dr Henery's legal and just claim, or submit to exposure of your filthy case.

Unfortunately for Wray and Anderson, Clarke was of the 'publish and be damned' calibre.

Wray tried to avoid the police court by taking to his bed and holding a pocket handkerchief to his mouth (and presumably doing a 'sick voice', though this detail is not recorded). After a policeman pulled the blankets off him, he said he had ignored the summons sent to Dr Henery on the grounds that he was not called Dr Henery. Wray was convicted at the Old Bailey of conspiracy to defraud and sentenced to two years' imprisonment. Anderson had a violent attack of delirium tremens after a few dry days in the house of detention but he, too, was tried and convicted. Patients like Clarke might have kept unscrupulous practitioners in business but they could also show the courage and determination to engineer their downfall.

Captain Clarke had eventually managed to get sensible advice from a qualified doctor, but orthodox treatments for spermatorrhoea could make the likes of Dr Henery seem a preferable option.

As a first resort, William Acton advocated giving up masturbation and seeing if the problem resolved itself, but in more severe cases, he recommended cauterisation. The patient was required to stand against a wall with a towel between his legs 'in order to protect the trowsers'. The surgeon would insert into the urethra a tube, on the end of which was a robust glass syringe containing a solution of nitrate of silver.

The piston of the instrument is then to be forced down, at the same time that the finger and thumb of the operator's left hand compress the lips of the meatus firmly against the instrument, so as to prevent the fluid escaping from the urethra until the syringe is withdrawn, which is done as soon as the injection has been forced out of the instrument.

The immediate result would be 'a warm pricking sensation at the end of the penis, which soon, however, subsides'. After resting in an armchair for a quarter of an hour and holding a handkerchief to the affected part for a bit longer, the patient was allowed to go home, but 'must not walk at all that day', even in the unlikely event that he felt any desire to do so. Acton asserted that the pain of this procedure was generally 'much less than the patient anticipated' but it is no surprise that many men preferred to try their luck with a vitalising belt from a newspaper advertisement.

Even doctors who avoided such aggressive treatments did not always inspire confidence. Francis Burdett Courtenay criticised those who, rather than get involved with such an unsavoury condition, dismissed the patient's concerns. One of his patients, the victim of a quack firm, had initially visited an eminent physician, only to be treated with impatience and indifference, handed a prescription and told: 'There, take that for six weeks, and if it does not do you any good, I don't know what will.' Courtenay reminded his medical readers that, tedious though patients' stories might be, it was a doctor's duty to 'submit with patience, taking the rough and smooth with equal equanimity'. If doctors chucked patients out after five minutes of refusing to believe them, they could hardly be surprised when swindlers fulfilled the human need to be heard and helped.

After his release from prison, Wray settled down to run a pub, but soon went back to his old ways, posing as Dr Albert Bell of Volta House, Wardour Street, whose Patent Voltaic

Belt would recover 'Health, Strength and Manly Vigour WITHOUT THE AID OF MEDICINE.' He died in 1890, leaving a nefariously collected fortune of £1,152 11s. In 1896, Dr Bell was summoned to court for using the titles M.D. and Doctor without being a qualified practitioner. On his name being called, there was no answer. The magistrate asked if the defendant was present and received the reply, 'No, Sir, he has been dead several years.'

HE WHO CAN HUMBUG BEST
IS THE CLEVEREST MAN

One of the occupational hazards of being a piss-prophet is that there's always some wise guy trying to take the … well, you know.

By the early nineteenth century, the diagnosis of disease by observing changes in the colour, consistency, smell and taste of urine had fallen into disrepute. Once a mainstream practice central to the methods of university-educated physicians, uroscopy gravitated to the fringes of the medical marketplace and the practitioner found himself derided by doctors as a 'water-quack' or 'piddle-taster'. Although professional physicians still acknowledged that taking note of the urine's condition could be a useful part of diagnosis, this was only alongside other diagnostic tools such as physical examination and taking a history. Their objection to the 'piss-prophets' was that these practitioners claimed to diagnose via urine alone, even in the patient's absence.

The late eighteenth century saw the publication of vehement denouncements of uroscopy, most notably John Coakley Lettsom's condemnation of the German practitioner Theodor Myersbach. Inspiring heated discussion about the merits or otherwise of Myersbach's methods, the debate widened awareness of the inefficacy of urine-casting, but by no means eradicated the practice.

48

Uroscopy's long history was difficult to erase and trust in it as a diagnostic method lingered among the general public. Perhaps the day-to-day effects of diet and hydration on urine's appearance helped to perpetuate its acceptance, for the belief was still going strong thirty years after Lettsom's publication, when Duncan Forbes M.D. asserted that:

> The vulgar regard the urine as a mirror in which all the internal operations of the body are immediately perceptible. They therefore expect that the physician, from the bare inspection of this excrementitious fluid, and disregarding every other symptom, should not only ascertain the nature of the disease, but also decide on the patient's constitution.

To set up as a 'water-doctor', there was no need to impose new beliefs on a credulous public, but simply to give them what they expected and demanded. Dr Cameron of Berners Street, off London's Oxford Street, embarked on this course during the first decade of the nineteenth century and was able to make a living by it for at least fifteen years. 'No surer method,' his adverts read, 'can be found to ascertain the nature and cause of Inward Complaints, than by inspecting and analysing the urine. It is by a sedulous study of this important discharge and its various changes and relations, that after an experience of twenty-five years, Dr Cameron has been enabled to perform cures when the first names and abilities in the profession have failed.'

Cameron's origins are obscure but the *Family Oracle of Health* presented him as a former apothecary called 'Coggins, or Crumples, or some such vulgar name', whose ignorance lost him his business and introduced the necessity of earning a crust in a more inventive way. Another account has him beginning his medical career by sharing premises in Wells Street with a silhouette-maker, advertising by employing a boy to stand at the street corner with a placard featuring Doctor Cameron on one side and a silhouette on the other.

In 1815, Cameron ditched his impoverished artist friend and moved round the corner to his own premises at Berners Street, still advertising by placard but venturing into the press too. Here, his proximity to the Middlesex Hospital enabled him to include its name in his adverts, at first using it to give directions to his house but later representing it as part of the address, perhaps hoping to form an associ-ation in the reader's mind between him and the respected institution.

Patients brought their morning urine – probably the whole lot, as quantity was a consideration – for Cameron to observe and taste before making a diagnosis and prescribing treatment. Although sweet-tasting urine had for centuries been recognised as an indicator of diabetes mellitus, Cameron's critics deemed him 'quite guiltless of all such knowledge'.

Rather like fortune-tellers, water-doctors were more successful when they could glean information from their patients and present it back to them. One method of doing this was to have a maidservant going about her daily work in the waiting room, listening out for any snippets of useful information as the patients chatted about their ailments. She could then convey this to the doctor just before the punter went in.

Cameron was known for the practice of 'chamber-puffing', or priming the patients in his waiting room to be receptive to his advice. For this he employed talkative people to pose as other patients and engage the real patients in conversation, saying that they were suffering from the same thing but that the doctor's treatment had already worked wonders.

In 1819, a letter appeared in the *Monthly Gazette of Health* suggesting that Cameron ran his water-tasting business as a secret sideline to the more mainstream occupation of apothecary. Jane Jones of Deptford had 'been an invalid forty-five years next December, and has been a pretty annuity to our family apothecary for that time', wrote her husband. Having been suffering with headaches and not gaining any benefit from six draughts a day of the apothecary's medicine, Mrs Jones saw the advertisement of a water-doctor in Berners Street and determined to consult him. The next morning the elderly couple travelled by stage the 6 or so miles to Charing Cross and 'toddled together' the rest of the way.

There they were admitted by a liveried servant and James Jones commented to his wife, 'Well, this looks well.' They were further reassured by what they later discovered were the 'chamber-puffers' and became even more well-disposed towards the doctor when a servant told them he would see them ahead of the other patients on account of their apparent fatigue.

'The doctor was sitting at a table well-loaded with books, with a wig, which inspired confidence and profound respect,' reported Mr Jones. 'My good old dame, who is never backward on such occasions, opened the business.' Mrs Jones told the doctor all about her symptoms and how the local apothecary wasn't doing her any good. It was only then that the doctor spoke and she recognised his voice. She looked closely and saw that beneath the wig was the very apothecary who had been attending her in Deptford for more than twenty years. Mr Jones was speechless: '"Well, well!" said I at last, "what a world we live in! All is humbug; and he who can humbug best is the cleverest man."' The doctor beseeched the Joneses 'in a most feeling manner' not to tell anyone at home about his alternative career.

Cameron is not named in the letter and it is, of course, possible that more than one water-doctor resided in Berners Street. Mr Jones, however, while clearly stating his own real name, made a point of signing his letter 'J. P. Cameron', indicating that this was a sort of in-joke with his wife. The *Medical Adviser* backs up the story by having its satirical portrayal of Cameron say: 'I am the physician of London one day, and the Deptford apothecary the next; thus keeping the mill hot, as it were.'

Dr Cameron's professed areas of expertise included liver disease, asthma and other lung conditions, dropsy, dysentery and 'the various complaints peculiar to females at the change of life'. At times he also advertised his ability to cure 'a Certain Disease', i.e. syphilis and all its complications – including 'gleets, strictures, diseased prostrate [sic] gland, and other alarming maladies of the generative organs'.

Cameron, no stranger to secrecy if the Joneses story is anything to go by, promised the utmost discretion in all cases. Patients too embarrassed or too incapacitated to attend in person had the option of sending a flask of urine (plus payment) via a messenger and receiving a written diagnosis and medicines in return. This system was a gift to pranksters and Cameron joined a long line of water-doctors falling foul of trickery. For all the popularity of 'piss-prophets', they also attracted those determined to challenge their skills – either out of revenge for unsatisfactory treatment or just for a laugh.

In 1778, Johann Georg Zimmermann related the case of a man who was pondering whether to consult a urine-caster and, having been ribbed about it, decided to send a mixture of urine, tincture of saffron and chalk. In return, he received a detailed account of the imaginary patient's illness and the method of cure, which convinced him not to bother asking the sender's advice about his own health.

Lettsom's investigation of Myersbach revealed similar stories. The German had allegedly mistaken Lisbon wine and elderflower water for a woman's urine and interpreted the products of a cow's bladder as belonging to someone who 'had been too free with the ladies of the town'.

Cameron's dose of horseplay came at the hands of a Holborn innkeeper whom he treated for chest pain. After a month of taking the prescribed pills, the patient became unable to urinate and, in agony in the middle of the night, had to send for a surgeon to catheterise him. The surgeon suspected that Cameron's pills, containing the purgatives jalap and calomel (mercurous chloride), were responsible for this unhappy episode. The innkeeper was determined on revenge.

His story was related by the *Medical Adviser*, which was so indignant in its ongoing campaign against quackery that it sometimes printed satirical fiction with well-known practitioners in the starring roles. The publication probably had no qualms about embellishing the details of this anecdote for the sake of entertainment, but claimed to have received them from a respectable source.

The innkeeper sent his ostler, along with a 'heavy' for back-up, to take a urine specimen to Cameron – a specimen that filled a quart bottle.

The doctor tasted the urine and concluded that the sufferer was in a bad way, but could be cured. By asking questions about the age of the patient (24), how hard he worked (lots of heavy loads) and whether he was a drinker (a pail of water twice a day), Cameron diagnosed a bad back, at which point the ostler revealed that the urine was from his donkey:

> "Get out of my house, you rascal!" bellowed the enraged "Doctor" as he chased the little ostler about the parlour, who now got behind his colossal assistant, and as well might Cameron pierce the shield of Ajax as make an impression upon him, so he contented himself with snatching up the bottle, opening the window and dashing it into the street.

He continued to rage at the visitors until they 'coolly retired'.

By 1824, Cameron's business was on the decline. His advertisements petered out of the newspapers and sunk away

THE QUACK DOCTOR

from the notice of the anti-quackery publications, whose contempt had perhaps hastened their departure.

'In the name of the north and the honor of old Scotland,' wrote the *Medical Adviser*, 'is this fellow a Cameron? And has the name that is associated with deeds of glory and the might of auld lang syne, dwindled into a filthy water-taster?'

7

TO RAISE FALSE HOPES

'Tears and prayers are of no use,' warned the eyecatching pictorial advertisement in the *Penny Illustrated Paper*. It was perhaps the most truthful statement Arthur Lewis Pointing, proprietor of Antidipso, had ever come up with.

Or rather, that the advertiser of a famous American anti-drunkenness medicine had ever come up with, for Pointing had lifted the copy verbatim. Pointing, a Londoner, had joined the Alaska Gold Rush after a court case put paid to his plans to convince short people that he could make them taller. His return to London in 1899 saw him bereft of gold but in possession of enough brass neck and stolen advertising copy to make his fortune. A decade later, he was worth almost £40,000 (equivalent to more than £3 million today). Unfortunately, he was no longer around to enjoy it, having met an end so unpleasant that no known remedy in the world could have saved him.

Born at Stoke Newington in 1867, Arthur Pointing gained some basic education before becoming a shop boy in his teens. In his early twenties he went into partnership with a German immigrant named Moritz Emil Kreyssig as a glass manufacturer, but after the business folded and a stint as head of a recruitment agency for housekeepers, ladies' companions and governesses also failed to pay off, Pointing's intact entrepreneurial spirit drew him into the world of dubious but not-quite-fraudulent advertising: 'ARE YOU LITTLE?'

asked the advertisements promoting the 'A. D. Invisible Elevators' from the Oriental Toilet Company. For 3*s* 9*d*, the elevators promised to increase anyone's height by up to 4 inches.

Enough people were curious enough to try them, for in the three months leading up to August 1897, Pointing made about £600. By this time, however, enough people had also realised that they were still as short as ever and so Inspector Leach of the Met went to have a quiet word.

When Pointing was arrested for fraud, the truth about the elevators rose to public view. At his hearing at Bow Street Police Court and subsequent trial at the Old Bailey, annoyed customers came forward to present their experiences.

Frederick Dry, an india-rubber worker and amateur actor from Manchester, replied to an advertisement and received promotional literature. With some scepticism, yet keen to look taller on stage, he sent off 3*s* 9*d*. Mr Dry testified:

> I got two pieces of cork, which I put in my boots, following the directions – they appeared to increase my height about one-eighth of an inch – I kept them there for about sixty minutes – they threw my body forward, and gave me a pain in the back, and cramped my toes – I took them out.

Other witnesses' evidence shows that it would be unwise to perceive them as vain or gullible for purchasing the product. Emily Turner of Upper Holloway hoped the elevators would provide a suitable alternative to the surgical boot she had been wearing since an injury to one of her legs. Sarah Trunnard from Leeds had in her care a little girl who had one leg shorter than the other and could only walk with the use of mobility apparatus. Mrs Trunnard had no expectation that her young charge would be cured, but did think the elevators might strengthen her.

When the elevators turned up, these small cork wedges backed with red paper proved useless – the little girl couldn't walk in them at all so Mrs Trunnard sent for her money back. But getting a refund out of the Oriental Toilet Company required determination of gigantic proportions.

When a potential customer enquired about the elevators, he or she would receive a circular sympathising with the plight of short people, who inevitably found themselves 'decried and treated with a certain amount of contempt and pity'.

'Many,' it said, 'will certainly speak in praise of little women, but few of little men.' This did not, however, mean that women didn't need the product:

> Little women, provided they are beautifully proportioned and know how to dress daintily, can be, and are, very attractive; but when these little women get past their fresh beauty and become fat or thin their trials begin. We all know how ridiculous it is to see a little fat woman waddling along like a motherly old duck, whereas a tall, stout, middle-aged woman does not look ridiculous at all.

After placing an order, most customers would receive a letter saying that the 3s 9d elevators were out of stock, but a superior version could be had on remittance of a further 1s 9d. If the customer asked for a refund instead, the elevators would arrive anyway. A proportion of customers probably decided at this point not to throw good money after bad and repurposed the cork wedges as doorstops in disgust, but persistent complainants met with further hurdles.

In lieu of a refund, they were offered a selection of toiletries, but even this was not all it seemed. Stephen Gent, a plumber from Burnley, agreed to receive a hand mirror for his daughter, but got a box of pills instead. If you wanted your 3s 9d back that much, you really had to work for it.

Staff of the Oriental Toilet Company revealed that the business address – 87, Strand – was unoccupied. A porter collected the post each day and took it to premises at Westminster Bridge Road, where employees sent out the replies. The company promoted additional products under various names and addresses, including a bust enlarger ostensibly sold by 'Madame E.P'.

Charlotte Smith, head clerk at Westminster Bridge Road, gave evidence that many customers were so satisfied with the elevators that they placed repeat orders. Pointing had told her that he might give up advertising as the profit was so small, but she had encouraged him to continue. He paid his staff's wages and his rent on time and if any complainants turned up, she dealt with them without Pointing's input.

The judge ruled that the Oriental Toilet Company was a genuine business and a few dissatisfied customers didn't warrant a conviction for fraud. Arthur Pointing was free, but the chances of anyone buying his Invisible Elevators had now shrunk to nothing. It was time to leave Oriental opportunities behind and go West.

The demise of the elevator business coincided with news that them there hills of Yukon, unlike the streets of London, were paved with gold. The 30-year-old Pointing set sail across the Atlantic to join the Klondike stampede.

Like most prospectors, he did not hit pay dirt. At least, not in any conventional way involving physical hardship and snow and things. While travelling across the U.S., however, he could not help but notice the money to be made in the patent medicine trade and the appropriately named Dr Haines's Golden Specific was one of the widely advertised remedies that caught his eye.

Products such as the Golden Specific, Magic Foot Drafts and the Thermal Vapor Bath Cabinet filled American newspapers' advertising columns with promises to cure all known illnesses.

Pointing wrote off for products and, instead of bemoaning the resulting flood of junk mail, carefully filed it away. He returned to London with a plan to replicate it and within just a few years had at least eight business concerns on the go. But, by then, a spirochaete bacterium was doing a little replication of its own – inside Pointing's body.

One of the most prominent of his products was also the most morally disconcerting. 'Antidipso', inspired by Dr Haines's Golden Specific, claimed to cure the most unregenerate drunkard. Said to be a natural remedy derived from little-known South American herbs, it had 'shed its radiance into thousands of hitherto desolate homes' and claimed to have 'guided many a young man to sobriety and into the high road of fortune'.

The number of unregenerate drunkards prepared to send off for a remedy was, of course, limited, so Antidipso was targeted at a more lucrative market – the drinker's loved ones. Enticing enquirers with a booklet called *Bright Beams of Hope*, Pointing – trading as the Ward Chemical Company – promised an end to day after day of lies, debt and vomit in the carpet. There need be no confrontation, no violence, no broken promises – a powder in the drinker's coffee would do the job in secret. The unsuspecting patient would be restored to the wholesome and sober bosom of his family and would once again become a man presentable enough for business success and social acceptance. The intended purchaser of Antidipso was not gullible; she was desperate.

The gendered language here is representative of the advertisements' assumptions. Although Pointing's ads sometimes acknowledged the possibility of female alcohol addiction, the character of the drinker was almost always presented as male. His saving angel, meanwhile, was a woman – usually a wife but perhaps a mother, sister or daughter. One advert, headlined 'HER FATHER WAS A DRUNKARD',

DRUNKENNESS CURED

It is now within the reach of Every Woman to
Save the Drunkard—A Free Trial Package
of a Marvellous Home Remedy
Posted to All Who
Write for it.

Can be Given in Tea, Coffee, or Food, thus absolutely and secretly Curing the Patient in a Short Time without his knowledge.

THERE is a cure for drunkenness which has shed a radiance into
thousands of hitherto desolate firesides. It does its work so
silently and surely that while the devoted wife, sister, or
daughter looks on, the drunkard is reclaimed even against his
will and without his knowledge or co-operation. The Company
who have this grand remedy will send a sample free to all
who will write for it. Enough of this remedy is posted in
this way to show how it is used in tea, coffee, or food, and
that it will cure the dreaded habit quietly and permanently.

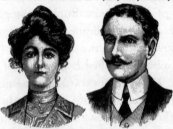

A lady residing in Manchester used the remedy as described
above, and her experience, told in her own words, will quite
likely interest all women deeply. Mrs.—— says: "Yes,
I used Antidipso without my husband's knowledge and
completely cured him. He was a hard drinker, a good man
when sober, but for years I lived in fear and dread, shame and
despair, poverty and disgrace. How shall I tell other women
about it? Is it not a wonderful thing that a woman can
take matters in her own hands and stamp out this dreadful
curse to the home? I am glad you are going to publish my
experience, for then I know it will reach hundreds of other
poor souls, and they will cure their husbands just as I cured
mine. I am so grateful for the marvellous changes that
have come into my life that I just feel like I would do anything
to let every wife and mother know what a blessing Antidipso
is. I honestly believe it will cure any drunkard, no matter
how far down he may have fallen.—Faithfully yours, Mrs.——."
(Full address sent to *bonâ-fide* applicants.)

Hundreds of others are reported, even the worst cases where
the habit seems to have blotted out the last remaining spark of
self-respect. Tears and prayers are of no use. Pleading,
pledges, loss of social or business position are unavailing to
stem the tide of absolute depravity.

This famous remedy has re-united thousands of scattered
families; it has saved thousands of men to social and business
prominence and public respect; has guided many a young man
into the right road to fortune; has saved the father, the
brother, the son, and in many cases the wife and daughter too.
Such a godsend to the home should be known to everyone.
Upon application to the WARD CHEMICAL CO., 9, CENTURY
HOUSE, REGENT STREET, LONDON, W., they will post a free
package of the remedy to you, securely sealed in a plain
wrapper, also full directions how to use it, books, testimonials
from hundreds who have been cured, and everything needed to
aid you in saving those near and dear to you from a life of
degradation and ultimate poverty and disgrace. Send for a
free trial to-day. It will brighten the rest of your life.

Antidipso.
*Author's
collection*

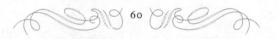

told the story of a plucky young lady who had set out to cure her dad – and, of course, succeeded.

Exhorted to 'take the matter into her own hands', the woman on the periphery of the alcoholic's life was presented with the alluring prospect of regaining some control over her situation – a situation that she could not escape, but might just be able to change. Testimonials told of wives who 'lived in fear and dread, shame and despair, poverty and disgrace', using Antidipso to regain the pleasant and hard-working men they thought they had married. In luring the alcoholic's wife with promises of a cure, Antidipso not only propagated false hope but also assigned to women responsibility for male behaviour: 'The poor drunkard is less able to take care of himself than an innocent prattling child. To do good by stealth is enjoined on us by the highest authorities.'

Helpless in his inebriated state, the man appears a passive victim of the demon drink, redeemed only by the pure and loving motives of a woman. She must adopt the role of guardian angel and mother to an infantilised abdicator of responsibility – it is up to her to change him and any failure will be her fault.

Bright Beams of Hope gave a history of Antidipso that shared characteristics with the promotion of other proprietary remedies of the late Victorian and Edwardian eras and which have not yet died out. While the medical profession was failing to cure alcholism, 'an obscure tropical plant was yielding the very remedy that acts as an antidote and expels the alcoholic poison'. The pamphlet assured its readers that the medicine was purely vegetable – an untainted, harmless product with its roots quite literally in nature. Discovered by an unnamed English physician, it had reached the notice of the Ward Chemical Company, who sent their own adventurer to verify it and bring it back to the drunkards of Britain.

To add gravitas to the product's credentials, the pamphlet reproduced a certificate from A.B. Griffiths, Principal of the Brixton School of Pharmacy, confirming that Antidipso had a 'marked therapeutic action'. Griffiths' name crops up in other patent medicine advertisements of the era and he regularly appeared in *Truth's Cautionary List* as someone prepared to give any remedy a good report on receipt of one guinea.

In 1904, representatives of the *British Medical Journal* replied to an Antidipso advertisement to see what would happen. They received a copy of *Bright Beams of Hope* and once on the mailing list could not escape the Ward Chemical Company's persistent exhortations to buy its product. 'You will not forget,' urged the literature, 'that to insure an absolute complete and permanent cure for the craving, two boxes are invariably required.'

The initial mailing was closely followed by an order form, and a third letter assured the enquirer that recent reports ('recent' being 1899, five years earlier) showed that, actually, a single packet would cure most patients. The prospective purchaser could even get a free supply of Antidipso by becoming an agent for the company, which involved buying in bulk and trying to convince all your friends that they were in need of a drunkenness cure. The next letter offered the product at half price.

The surreptitious nature of the treatment was not just marketing hyperbole – the product itself was designed for concealment. When the British Medical Association acquired a packet for analysis in 1904, they discovered that the powders, though similar in composition, came in two colours – the purchaser could choose the most appropriate one depending on the colour of the food or drink to be laced. *The Lancet* noted the concealed nature of the treatment with disgust, asserting:

Century Thermal
Bath Cabinet.
Author's collection

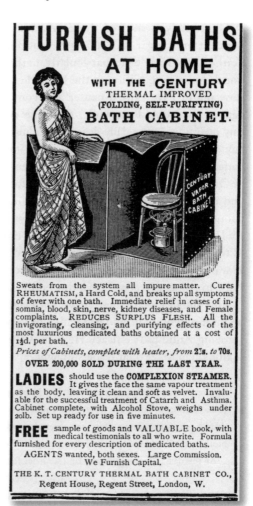

There have been many cruel and wicked frauds committed by the
sellers of quack medicines but of all that have come to our notice we
do not know one of a baser character than that which is perpetrated
by the proprietor of antidipso.

Their analysis showed the product to comprise 78.22 per cent milk sugar and 21.78 per cent potassium bromide, neither of which were particularly herbal or particularly South American. Although the bromide in a large enough dose might have caused nausea and vomiting, putting the patient off alcohol for a while, *The Lancet* concluded that the tiny quantities in the daily dose of Antidipso would not make any difference. Even a placebo effect was impossible since the patient was unaware he was under treatment.

One packet of Antidipso, comprising forty-eight powders and retailing at 10*s*, contained ingredients to the value of about 1½*d*. The large mark-up, however, was of little concern to *The Lancet* reporter, who thought that 'if people are so silly as to buy quack remedies they must expect to pay for them'. It was the coldheartedness of the whole scheme, raising false hope in vulnerable people, that the reporter found scandalous.

After publication of these views, *The Lancet*'s offices received a visit from Pointing, who had with him a sheaf of testimonials 'proving' Antidipso's efficacy. He then wrote to them politely asking them to set their readers straight.

> You read letters from patients themselves blessing the day that they took Antidipso; you have letters from mothers, wives and sisters thanking us for putting within their reach the means of curing their brothers, husbands, and fathers of the craving for drink.
>
> All this data fully warrants the claim we make for this specific …

To Pointing, the word 'data' did not mean what everybody else thought it meant.

The Ward Chemical Company operated out of 203 Regent Street in London, impressive premises that still stand today. Sharing this accommodation was the Century Thermal Bath Cabinet Company, which offered the health benefits of a steam bath in the comfort of one's own parlour. Set up in 1899, the company sold portable wooden compartments that could be erected around a chair and a basin of boiling water to create a steam room. This innovation, a convenient and private alternative to visiting a proper Turkish bath and trekking home in the cold, was such a hit with the public that within four years the business had expanded to employ seventy people and had agents as far afield as Australia and South Africa. Its managing director was, of course, the ubiquitous Arthur Lewis Pointing.

Such baths were not without their dangers. Just after Christmas in 1903, 21-year-old Bertha Pollard was burnt to death when she knocked over the lamp supplying the heat to her bath and could not escape from the flammable wooden compartment surrounding her. The coroner took a dim view of the sale of these devices, saying it was 'highly reprehensible' to put them on the market.

Tragedies like this were rare, however, and thermal baths remained in vogue long enough to make Arthur Pointing's fortune. And not only did he sell bath cabinets and drunkenness cures, but operated at least six other businesses capitalising on people's desire to be healthy and beautiful. There was the Espanola Medicine Company, whose Diano product promised to increase women's bust size by 6 inches: 'Diano has a wonderful effect,' read a testimonial from one Mrs Crook, 'Bosoms are getting quite full.' Hirsute people could choose from the Helen Temple Depilatory or Capillus, another hair destroyer that claimed, 'Hairy women need no longer despair'. The Fell Formula, which comprised milk sugar and extract of bladderwrack (a common component of proprietary obesity pills), promised weight loss of a whopping 7lb a day. There were also the Murray Company (which offered artificial ear drums to cure hearing loss of any cause) and the Grecian School of Physical Culture, described by *Truth* as 'a reproduction of a Yankee notion for teaching physical exercises by correspondence'.

But however much money these ventures made for Pointing, it was not enough to save him from the bacteria that had colonised his brain. It is impossible to say at what point in his eventful career Pointing contracted syphilis, but the devastating tertiary stage of the disease took hold when he was at the height of his success.

In October 1905, he was taken ill in the street. Within a few days, he was back at business at Century House and a month later was enjoying a round of golf in Brighton with his friend, the advertising agent Thomas Platt. But his recovery was only temporary. He was showing signs of general paralysis of the insane, a neurological condition resulting from syphilitic infection and resembling severe psychiatric symptoms.

On 26 July 1906, when he was 38, Pointing's mental health broke down irretrievably and he was removed to Peckham House Asylum on Camberwell Road. No records survive of his four-year stay there, but in common with other GPI patients he would have experienced delusions, progressive dementia, seizures and loss of muscular function, ending up paralysed and doubly incontinent. This living death became a merciful one on 14 April 1910. Pointing was 42 years old and left a fortune of £37,909 2s 6d, some of which he specified should go to his employees and some to charity.

If *The Lancet* were capable of influencing people's fate, it might be said to have done so when it opined of Antidipso's proprietor: 'To raise false hopes in those whose lot it is to be tied to a drunkard is disgraceful and no punishment can be too bad for the person who profits by such deceit.' Even *The Lancet*, however, could surely not have been heartless enough to revel in the nature of Arthur Lewis Pointing's demise.

8

A LONG LIFE AND A BUSY ONE

The grotesque humanoid form of the mandrake root, screaming fatally when ripped from the earth, has inspired tales of the supernatural from Josephus to J.K. Rowling. In the 1890s, however, Joshua Barrett became a down-to-earth Mandrake Specialist whose success relied less on magic than on hard work, enthusiasm and a peculiar portrait of himself pretending to be a duck.

Go to any twenty-first-century country show, craft fair or exhibition and chances are you'll see at least one stall flogging health products that 'can help with' whatever happens to be wrong with you. Barrett used the same method to sell his Mandrake Embrocation and subsidiary products designed to cure every ailment of human, horse, or dog. He travelled far and wide with his exhibition stand and its sign promising passers-by: 'I will cure, in one minute, headache, earache, or toothache, free of charge. I wish by this means to prove to the public the value of my marvellous mandrake embrocation.'

Barrett came from a respected Baptist family that farmed in St Ives, Huntingdonshire. He began his career as a warehouseman in the lace industry, later becoming a travelling salesman in drapery. It was in the late 1880s, however, that he went into the patent medicine trade, moving to Islington and promoting Barrett's Mandrake Embrocation for sprains, bruises, overstraining of the muscles, cramp, rheumatism, sciatica, lumbago, gout, neuralgia and fits, as well as the ailments mentioned on his sign. A few drops of embrocation rubbed on the forehead would stop a headache instantly and at the Morley Hall Bazaar, Hackney, in 1888, Barrett claimed to have cured twenty people right there and then. Whether bazaars were a particular congregating ground for people with headaches, he did not elucidate.

The most striking thing about Barrett's marketing was his registered trademark, a visual pun on the word 'mandrake' that showed the likeness of Barrett's head, complete with top hat, attached to the body of a drake. Described as 'bizarre' by the *Chemist and Druggist*, this frightening coalition of salesman and anatid attracted curious people to Barrett's exhibition stand and was also embossed on the Embrocation bottles themselves.

When the Russian influenza pandemic reached the UK in late 1889, Barrett was quick to add the disease to the list of those powerless against the Embrocation. He had not so far promoted his product as a treatment for flu, but as outbreaks raged across the globe, the Embrocation became 'Scientifically Proved and Practically Demonstrated' as a cure. Handbills explained why flu had never been mentioned before: 'This remedy has only just been discovered, and the following directions are not with the Thousands of Bottles now in the hands of the appreciative public.'

The symptoms of the strain of flu that iced the surface of the world in 1889 were as miserable as can be imagined. William Gordon Stables, the writer of adventure fiction who was also a doctor and author of *The People's ABC Guide to Health*, described the onset of the disease as so sudden that it could strike people in the middle of eating their dinner.

> There is decided chilliness, and sometimes even shivering. The headache and feeling of oppression, and tightness across the brow,

are often very great. Sneezing is another troublesome symptom, with running of water, both from the eyes and nose, the eyelids being sometimes very much swollen.

Sufferers could also expect a racking cough, dry throat, furred tongue, tight chest and a feeling of physical weakness accompanied by great depression of spirits. The latter was not to be underestimated. Luton photographer Harry Creasy shot himself dead after the Russian flu left him weakened and depressed, while Police Constable Islip of the Croydon force was removed to Cane Hill Asylum when the virus seriously 'affected his mind'. Nausea, vomiting and diarrhoea were more common and a cold sweat would overtake the person's aching body.

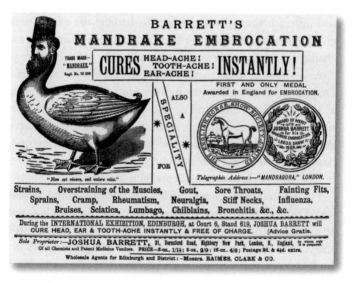

Barrett's Mandrake Embrocation. *Image © Bodleian Library, University of Oxford 2008: John Johnson Collection, Patent Medicines 1 (33). Copyright © 2008 ProQuest LLC. All rights reserved*

The majority of otherwise healthy people, however, would recover from influenza after around a week. It was a smart move for patent medicine proprietors to recommend their product as flu specific – most purchasers would indeed feel better within a few days of taking it.

To ward off the early symptoms of flu, Barrett advised his customers to 'take a piece of sponge the size of an egg, damp with the Embrocation, and hold it to the open mouth, inhale steadily, then close the mouth, swallow the fumes, and return them through the nostrils: repeat often'. Although an egg-sized piece of sponge was adequate, Barrett also sold a special inhaler. A simple glass tube designed to hold an embrocation-soaked piece of wadding, it was cheap at only a shilling. In the more advanced stages of influenza, Barrett also advised rubbing the oil on all achey parts of the body. This was as good a treatment as any, although Gordon Stables's recommendation is hard to beat: 'To combat the prostration good wine will be required, or even brandy; but I think champagne will answer in most cases.'

At a show in 1890, a representative of the *Chemist and Druggist* chatted to Barrett, lightheartedly referring to him as the 'apostle of mandrake'. Although Barrett claimed to have cured seventeen people of toothache that day, he wasn't convinced that this would boost sales. 'In the south,' he said, 'when we cure a case of toothache, the relieved sufferer buys a bottle of our marvellous medicine; here he does not.'

He was confident, however, that the northern mind 'would come right in time'. Optimism prevailed and Barrett relocated to Gowdall Lane, Snaith, where his 'Mandrake House' still looks out over farmland today. His wife Margaret, to whom he had been married since 1874, does not appear to have accompanied him, staying in Islington and later being elected as a Poor Law Guardian – a position still unusual for women at that time. At some point Barrett employed a housekeeper,

Martha Ann Penty, who was to remain with him for the rest of his life.

From the Embrocation sprouted other remedies, including the Mandrake Liver Powder, of which a testimonial writer enthused: 'If all the world knew its value, all the world would use it.' Accounts of agricultural shows imply that Barrett also sold cures for the ailments of animals.

He could turn his hand to emergencies too. When a yearling colt kicked a man in the face at the Devon County Show in 1895, Barrett – who held an Ambulance Class first-aid certificate – patched up the wound. His 'conduct and skill on this occasion were highly spoken of'.

A 1908 handbill in the Bodleian Library's John Johnson Collection refers to 'Mandrake fields' in Bluntisham, suggesting that at the time Barrett was living in Snaith and doing the exhibition rounds, his ingredients were growing on the family farm. The contents of many patent medicines – and the honesty of their proprietors – turned out to be rather less than claimed, as the British Medical Association's analyses showed in the same year, but it is likely that the Mandrake Embrocation was a genuine herbal product in which Barrett himself had faith.

There is, however, mandrake and mandrake. During his days in London, Barrett had used the telegraphic address 'Mandragora' – the genus of the mandrake plant that, according to folklore, screamed on being uprooted, causing the death of whoever dared to rip it from the ground. His handbills also claimed that the author of *The Complete Herbalist*, O. Phelps Brown, 'says of "Mandrake" "In Chronic Liver Diseases it has no equal in the whole range of medicines"'.

Phelps Brown did give this opinion – but about the American mandrake plant, podophyllum, rather than Barrett's product. The quotation marks around 'Mandrake' are disingenuous, added by Barrett in order to present Phelps Brown's words

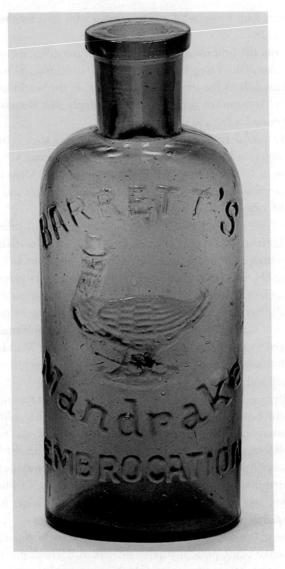

Barrett's Mandrake Embrocation bottle. *Reproduced by kind permission of Michael Till, www.michaeltill.com*

as an endorsement of the Embrocation. When the *Gardener's Chronicle* encountered him at the Sandy flower show in 1889, however, they were sceptical about the identity of the 'large root of white colour, resembling a huge, many-branched Beet' that adorned his stand. The *Chronicle's* representative believed it to be deadly nightshade, in whose genus, *Atropa*, mandrake had also been classified.

A hint as to the real contents of the Embrocation comes from later in Barrett's career, after he and Martha Penty had left Snaith for another newly christened Mandrake House in Beechfield Avenue, Blackpool. Barrett put a notice in the papers offering to pay 10*s* per hundredweight for freshly dug mandrake root. He specified, however, that by 'mandrake' he meant white bryony.

This plant, *Bryonia dioica*, had a history of being passed off as the real thing. Maud Grieve, in her *Modern Herbal* (1931), quoted Thomas Green's assertion from 1832 that imposters would fix human-shaped moulds around the growing roots, producing their very own 'mandrakes' for sale to the unsuspecting public. An alternative name for white bryony is 'the English mandrake' and Grieve refers to it being known as 'mandrake' in Norfolk – not a vast distance from Barrett's Huntingdonshire childhood home.

Bryony, though poisonous, was traditionally used as a purgative and laxative and was considered efficacious against dropsy. At the time of Grieve's writing, herbalists recommended the plant for lung complaints – including influenza.

It would, however, have been possible for Barrett's family to cultivate Mandragora in the climate of Bluntisham. There is a chance that he innocently considered the white bryony plant to be the genuine mandrake. But to have upheld his product as mandrake for decades in the face of public opinion suggests that he knew his botany. It is not inconceivable that the energetic salesman used Mandragora but shrewdly resorted to substitutes when supplies were low.

In 1919, Joshua Barrett finally married Martha Penty and they remained at Blackpool until his death in 1931 at the age of 81. The wish of a grateful punter, whom the Mandrake Embrocation relieved of a decade-long earache in 1898, had come true:

> Accept my very best thanks for your kindness, and may both yourself and Mandrake have a long life and a busy one.

9

THEY NEVER CAME OUT
OF THE HUMAN FOOT

It is a notorious fact that persons will cut their corns with razors, knives and other unwieldy instruments, as if their toes were not of any importance to the general system, or put themselves into the hands of any man who, with plausibility, would promise a radical cure, without thinking for one moment how soon an accident would deprive them of the power of taking exercise and disregarding the various results that might follow.

Lewis Durlacher (1792–1864), surgeon-chiropodist to Her Majesty Queen Victoria, lamented the public's tendency to dismiss foot problems, battling on with ill-fitting shoes and questionable hygiene until their corns were so painful that they would resort to hacking them about.

The medical profession (with exceptions such as Sir Benjamin Brodie, who lectured on the subject in 1836) was not very interested either, regarding corns as the province of itinerant corn-cutters pretentiously referring to themselves as 'chiropodists'. To them, there was something ludicrous in the long newspaper adverts of expensive practitioners such as the Polish chiropodist John Eisenberg, who printed unlikely testimonials from the nobility of Europe, including Emperor Napoleon III ('Monsieur Eisenberg m'a extrait les cors avec un grand success et une grande habilitè').

However rich and famous the sufferer, consulting a qualified chiropodist was not an option, for there were none. Lack of regulation left the unwary patient unable to differentiate between the most skilled and ethical practitioners – such as Durlacher – and those who were ineffective, dangerous or even fraudulent. Durlacher was outspoken about the need for regulation:

> From such men the public, being unable of themselves to distinguish between the competent practitioner and the empiric, ought to be protected either by legislative enactments, or by medical bodies licensing those who make chiropody a part of their regular medical education.

The professionalisation of chiropody was still a long way off – Europe's first Society of Chiropodists was not formed until 1912. But if someone was in agony with corns, they could hardly hang around waiting for the twentieth century to arrive. Thomas Ashton, House Surgeon at University College Hospital and later surgeon to the Blenheim Dispensary, illustrated the extent of sufferers' desperation with the case of a 20-year-old servant tormented by a corn on the little toe of her left foot. Unable to bear the pain any longer, she placed a knife-blade against the toe and struck it 'either with a cleaver or a mallet', sending both corn and toe into oblivion and leaving an exposed section of bone. 'Considerable haemorrhage occurred' and her mistress was alarmed enough to send her to hospital, where she eventually recovered.

The less determined must either treat their own corns, consult a surgeon or general practitioner who might or might not 'do feet', or employ someone with a reputation as a corn-cutter – some of whom were more skilled and honest than others. Paring one's own corns might have carried the danger of drawing blood and contracting septicaemia, but the additional risk with corn-cutters was being bled of large sums of cash.

An 1846 correspondent to *The Lancet* described how an earl of his acquaintance was fleeced by a chiropodist known to be preying on elderly wealthy customers. The earl, aged 78, had two troublesome corns and was so anxious to get rid of them that the corn-cutter's demand of 10s per corn seemed a reasonable deal.

> The operation commenced; when it was over, the corn-cutter presented my friend with a paper on which were arranged 116 corns, or dark somethings which he designated such, and smilingly announced his claim of £58!

The earl paid up and, 'inwardly cursing the chiropodist for a knave and himself for a fool', didn't admit the episode to his family for several weeks. When his wife had stopped laughing she took great delight in relating the tale to their doctor friend, who submitted it to *The Lancet*. His opinion on what he would have done in the same situation was: 'I would have made the fellow eat up his corns, and then kicked him down stairs.'

But how was it physically possible for a chiropodist to extract 116 corns from the earl's foot?

He was not alone in this remarkable ability, for his methods were common practice among the less reputable chiropodists of the time. *The Lancet* correspondent had been inspired to write in by the case of a German-born practitioner named Joseph Wolff, who had recently been tried for, and acquitted of, obtaining the sum of £1 from a Suffolk gentleman by false pretences. And five years before, a chiropody double-act, Messrs Rembrand and Nieman, had been committed to the Northleach House of Correction in Cheltenham in similar circumstances. The evidence given in court in both these cases provides an insight into the way corn-cutters reaped such a lucrative harvest.

Wolff initially approached Southwold doctor Robert Wake with a letter of recommendation from one of Wake's patients, suggesting that he introduce the chiropodist to other corn-sufferers. The endorsement appears to have been genuine and followed an operation in which Wolff extracted twenty-five corns for a fee of £6, which was a pretty impressive trick seeing as the patient only had four corns to start with. Accompanying the letter was a collection of convincing-looking certificates and testimonials from noblemen and eminent physicians. As Dr Wake himself was troubled by corns, he suggested that if Wolff successfully operated on them without charge, he would recommend his services. Prudently, Wolff extracted only four from Dr Wake's four visible corns.

Wake introduced him to his friend William Fonnereau, Esq, 'from whose feet the operator produced four, and from another member of the same family, eight spicula of the same horny, bristly or bony substance, some being smooth, some somewhat jagged, and some a little curved at the points'. On examining the first lot, Dr Wake finally cottoned on that something dodgy was afoot. He tried to observe the operation but Wolff complained that he was obstructing the light. In a letter to the main medical journals, Wake later described what he saw:

> With crooked scissors, of various sizes, having clipped away all uneven surfaces from the different corns under operation, then with a suitable solemnity the operator took from a round box a bottle of mysterious oil, somewhat resembling blood, which he represented as having the power to raise the corns. This oil was with abundant care rubbed over each toe operated upon, and into each excavation made in it, until it foamed; and at this perhaps critical period of the operation, the operator invariably resorted to some manoeuvre to attract the attention of the bystander, and each flap before spoken of being carefully closed over

the orifice, and the oil wiped from the outer part of the toes, the chiropodist then by means of an instrument, like a large silver toothpick, with great adroitness, disengaged what he called the corns, and brought them one by one to view, exclaiming – 'See de corn.' The object being thus made visible, the operator taking up a pair of long, broad forceps, deeply grooved, and closing with a slide, proceeded to lay hold of it, and suiting the action to the extremity of the case, he affected to exercise the utmost judgement and care in the ceremony of extraction, which, having with apparent difficulty effected, the self-created corn was usually triumphantly exhibited, and its point applied to the back of the patient's hand, no doubt that its power to give pain might be felt.

Rembrand and Nieman also made their living by extracting large numbers of 'somethings' from small numbers of corns. In October 1841, they appeared before the Cheltenham magistrates on a charge under the Vagrancy Act of 1824, which encompassed 'Every person pretending to or professing to tell fortunes, or using any subtle craft, means or device, by palmistry or otherwise, to deceive or impose upon any of her Majesty's subjects.' Chiropody, still far from acceptance as a health profession, came under the category of 'otherwise'.

Rembrand and Nieman, however, did not fit the stereotypical image of the vagrant. Despatched to bring them in, the police returned with 'a foreigner, dressed in the pink of fashion, who gave his name as Lee Rembrand. He was followed shortly after by another gaily-dressed young man, whose face was adorned with a pair of bushy whiskers and fine black moustachios. He said his name was Nieman.' Rembrand, who claimed to be chiropodist to the late King of Prussia, was the principal practitioner and Nieman the sidekick. They had allegedly charged a man called Charles Barker the sum of £8 15s for extracting thirty-five corns. After the operation, Mr Barker 'felt as much pain and pressure as before' and a corn-cutter at the Cheltenham Baths was of the opinion that nothing at all had been done. Barker asked a local chemist to consult Rembrand as a test, and this patient managed to get one of the 'corns' to take home as a curiosity. Another customer, Caroline Bradley, also managed to keep hold of the substances extracted from her feet, having convinced Rembrand that she wanted to show them to friends suffering a similar malady. In court, the evidence of a chemist and a surgeon narrowed down the corns' identity to either bristle, toenail or quill.

Five years later, Joseph Wolff explained the large quantity of 'somethings' by theorising that the bones of the feet constantly threw out painful spikes into the visible lesions designated corns. Dr Wake, however, became 'quite sure that they never came out of the human foot'. He and Mr Fonnereau enlisted amateur microscopist Reverend S. Clissold to identify the spicula. Mr Clissold believed them to be pieces of herring-bone.

Wolff, who had returned from Southwold to his home in Norwich, was arrested and tried at the Suffolk Christmas Sessions. In contrast to the dapper appearance of Rembrand and Nieman, the prisoner was 'dressed in a loose brown coat with a light waistcoat, had a fine intelligent countenance, but his appearance was not at all professional'.

Farrier William Blowers gave evidence that he had seen Wolff outside his father's forge, gathering up the parings of horses' hooves, the implication being that he had used them to create his patients' false corns. Whatever the nature of the spicula, however, either Mr Clissold or Dr Wake had managed to lose them, and there was not enough evidence to secure a prosecution.

It was not until thirty years later that Wolff's methods finally caught up with him. In 1877, the chiropodist, by then 66, was in Cambridge trying his luck at extracting corns and coins from wealthy students. They had more clout than the citizens of Southwold and he was convicted of obtaining the sum of 30*s* by false pretences from the Honourable John William Plunkett, son of Lord Dunsany. Wolff's own feet spent the next four months acquiring an in-depth knowledge of the prison treadmill.

10

DODGING ABOUT ALL
OVER ENGLAND

Miss Julia Opie was a young woman of very great respectability. A draper's assistant, she worked in Redruth with twenty other respectable young women for a highly respectable employer named Mr Corin. When her hearing began to deteriorate, she saw nothing untoward in answering an advertisement from a retired clergyman, the Reverend J. Johnstone of Heavitree in Somerset, who had cured himself of deafness and now wished to share his good fortune with the world.

The reply to her letter wasn't quite what she expected. As some might say of the deity to whom he professed allegiance, the Reverend Mr Johnstone did not exist and rather than some avuncular advice about deafness, Miss Opie received a 'filthy publication' written by one Baron McKinsey.

McKinsey was 'a herbalist who lives in some "style" at Heavitree'. He had been selling his botanical medicines for almost thirty years without much trouble, but once his *True Guide to Health* had aroused the moral indignation of Miss Opie's employer, his fortunes changed. Faced with imprisonment under the Obscene Publications Act, he took the only route open to the self-respecting accusé and legged it. The police, however, were not going to forget about him. It took nine years to find the Baron and bring him to trial.

Baron McKinsey's Katapotia – the name taken from an ancient Greek word for pills – arrived on the market in the mid-1840s, when their inventor was around 21 years old. Starting out as plain Henry McKinsey, he soon adopted the cognomen of 'Baron McKinsey M.D.' By the age of 30 he was claiming to have fourteen years' experience as a doctor, to have been a pupil of the celebrated Ernst Dieffenbach at Berlin and to have been Consulting Physician to the Hôpital Venerien in Paris.

The Katapotia, or Life-Preserving Pills, were a panacea, 'designated the most efficacious remedy extant for all diseases arising from a disorganisation of the stomach, bowels or liver, such as bilious and liver complaints, indigestion, constipation of bowels, debility, fevers, giddiness, headache, heartburn, jaundice, nervous affections, &c. &c.' Tapeworms were among the conditions powerless against the medicine's effects and in 1852 the Baron claimed to have expelled a creature more than 32 feet long from the bowels of Mr G. Reynolds of Dartmoor.

McKinsey operated two advertising methods concurrently. Lengthy advertisements celebrated the Katapotia's cures with lively testimonials such as the following from George Augustus Wood, J.P.:

Sir

I have derived more benefit from your invaluable Medicine than I have received FOR YEARS from physicians' prescriptions, and I have taken, I believe, as much physic as would have poisoned a troop of rhinoceros.

Less flashy, however, were the brief notices placed by 'The Rev J. Johnstone'. Often headlined 'For the Good of Suffering Humanity', they promised to forward the particulars of a cure for deafness and nose polyps on receipt of a stamped envelope. In 1856, a publication called the *Interview* sent off a stamp as

THE GLORY OF MAN IS STRENGTH.

BARON McKINSEY, Lecturer on Medical Botany, Physiology, Pathology, Anatomy, &c., author of the "Guide to Health, or every person his own Physician," which describes how the nervous and debilitated can be restored, and the vigour of manhood maintained to an advanced period of life, sent free by post on receipt of a postage stamp. Address—Baron McKinsey, European Institution and Anatomical Museum, Heavitree-park, near Exeter, Devon.

EDITORIAL NOTICE FROM THE LONDON TIMES —We have inspected several authentic letters testifying to the wonderful cures effected by Baron McKinsey, of Heavitree-park, Exeter, of Polypus and other complaints, which many of the most eminent of the Faculty have been unable to cure. The Baron has obtained a world-wide celebrity for his Medicines, which, in numberless cases have proved thoroughly efficac'ous in curing all manner of diseases. Should any of our readers be suffering from any sort of ailment. we advise them to apply to Baron McKinsey for the true Guide to Health.

Baron McKinsey's Botanical Preparations are the most scientifically prepared Medicines ever compounded by human skill. The Royal Patent Medicinal Powder is a certain cure for Polypus in the nose, Deafness, Defect of Sight, Fits, Apoplexies, and all diseases of the Head. —Sold in boxes at 2s 9d. The Katapotia, or Life Preserving Pills remove all oppressive accumulations, regulate the secretions of the liver and kidneys, strengthen the stomach, purify the blood, and prolong existence. —Sold in boxes at 1s. 1½d., and 2s. 9d., by all Medicine Vendors.

N.B.—Be sure you observe that each box has the words "Baron McKinsey, Heavitree-park," engraved on the Government Stamp.

Baron McKinsey's Botanical Preparations. *Sherborne Mercury, Tuesday 13 December 1864. Image © THE BRITISH LIBRARY BOARD. ALL RIGHTS RESERVED. Image reproduced with kind permission of the British Newspaper Archive (www.britishnewspaperarchive.co.uk)*

part of an investigation into newspaper advertisements and received in return a badly printed booklet mostly consisting of testimonials for Baron McKinsey's medicines.

The integrity of these testimonials was called into question at Hereford in 1860, when the Baron distributed pamphlets featuring an endorsement from M.A.C. Coldroodge of 4 Widemarsh Street, beseeching him to accept a thank you gift of a 'silver card, fruit or biscuit tray, which I shall send from hence by the G.W. express at eleven o'clock on Monday morning next, trusting it may be sufficiently approved of to ensure a corner amongst the bijouterie in the drawing room at Heaviside Park'. Coldroodge's presence was news to the people actually living at 4 Widemarsh Street, who were not in the habit of despatching bijouterie to fake barons.

Other than this 'little mistake' and the occasional 'mean, petty, envious, and ungenerous opinions' of detractors, McKinsey's business seems to have run fairly smoothly until 1874. In that year, the Baron had been using a testimonial purportedly sent to Exeter Police by an American keen to track down the wonderful remedies. But while it was appearing in the papers, the Exeter Police were getting far more involved than the Baron had bargained for.

By then Julia Opie had sought a cure for her hearing loss. Her employer, having ripped some pages from the *True Guide to Health* in disgust, had sent them to Exeter's Chief Constable, who had an unfortunate name for a copper – Captain Bent.

The pages' contents were filthy enough for Bent to investigate further, so he arranged for a letter to go to the Reverend J. Johnstone under the pseudonym of Miss Maria Willcocks of Plymouth, a young lady afflicted with partial deafness and nervousness. The reply contained the same booklet, and on going to Heaviside Park with a search warrant, Captain Bent and a colleague found a vast number of copies ready to be despatched.

The entire 9,000 of them were piled up in front of the bench at Exeter Castle when McKinsey was hauled in for a hearing. Opinion on their contents became emotive; Mr Friend, for the prosecution, stated that 'a more filthy, abominable, and immoral publication could scarcely be put into circulation, and the mere act of circulating it was assailing the privacy of every man's dwelling and striking at the very foundation of all domestic morality and happiness'. What on earth could be so offensive?

News reports of the trial were loath to propagate the vile texts and referred to them in vague terms designed to leave the morals of lady readers intact. They hinted, however, at chapters titled 'The Disappointed Bride' and 'The Charming Wife'. The Baron's advertisements give further clues as to the contents, indicating that among the multitude of conditions vanquished by the Katapotia were 'nervous and sexual debility, arising from excess or solitary indulgence, weakness, irregularity, impotency, loss of appetite, syphilis, barrenness, obstinate gleets, and all other urino-genital diseases'. The booklet contained 'remarks on the secret causes of self-acquired miseries and disappointed hopes' and advised on how the vigour of manhood could be maintained. In other words, the offensive material was something to do with willies and the various solo or companionable adventures thereof.

McKinsey's not unreasonable defence was that he intended the booklet as a medical treatise to educate people on how to maintain their health, and that it was no more offensive than the publications written by the eminent medical practitioners of the day.

Yet the issue of obscene publications was in the ether, with prosecutions hitting the headlines in London. In early 1873, John Davidson, the owner of Dr Kahn's anatomical museum, which displayed waxworks suitable for the eyes of 'gentlemen only', had been tried at the Old Bailey for

> "A wise physician, skilled our wounds to heal,
> Is more than armies to the public weal."

SUCH is the testimony of poetry to the national value of Medical Science. One wise, experienced and observant man, well acquainted with human maladies, and skilful in the application of natural and rational remedies, is of more service to the nation than legions of red coats and forests of bayonets. Let the wise and patriotic reflect upon this fact, and learn a lesson of political economy ; let the prejudiced reflect upon this fact, and learn that there are more things in heaven and earth than are dreamt of in our philosophy; let the educationist reflect upon this fact, and learn that national education will be incomplete until medical knowledge and physical training occupy a significant place in his formulæ. Let the sick and suffering add to their appreciation of this fact the knowledge which we can impart to them. We have had submitted to us, by grateful patients, a large number of extraordinary and unheard of cases performed by this wonderful man — some of those cases having been dismissed from public infirmaries as incurable. At first we received these testimonials with suspicion ; but truth is stronger than fiction, and after diligent attention and enquiry, we are compelled to confess that Baron McKinsey's system of medicine is the greatest discovery of the age. No disease seems capable of baffling his penetration and genius. Blindness and deafness, polypus in the nose, diseases of the head and chest, heart and lungs, stomach, liver and kidneys, all alike seem to be perfectly under his control ; and if we might make a selection we should say that in asthma, consumption, indigestion, rheumation, nervous debility, scrofula, scorbutic and other diseases, his success appears truly astounding. Those desirous of consulting him will find him at the European Institution, Heavitree Park, near Exeter. Entrance by the Lodge-gate, opposite the first mile stne on the Honiton-road from Exeter.

Baron McKinsey. *Sherborne Mercury, Tuesday 13 December 1864. Image*

publishing *The Philosophy of Marriage: an Exposition of the Duties and Responsibilities of Married Life*. In September the same year, George Essen and David MacDonald – the latter only 17 years old – were each sentenced to two years' hard labour for carrying on 'a very disgusting and nefarious business' in indecent literature and pictures. Could the Baron's case be a good opportunity for the Exeter Police to get in on the act?

McKinsey was defended by Mr Besley, who had for years been counsel to the Society for the Suppression of Vice and had acted for the prosecution in the Kahn case. He had seen a few obscene publications in his time and McKinsey's was nothing to get excited about. To him, the trial appeared to have more to do with Captain Bent's zeal – perhaps inspired by the London prosecutions – than with the actual content of the book.

McKinsey promised to expunge the objectionable passages from future editions, but this was not enough for the court, which condemned all copies of the book to destruction. The Baron intended to appeal. Before the Quarter Sessions came round, the appeal was abandoned, but Captain Bent and his officers decided that destroying the books was not sufficient punishment for this 'person of wicked and depraved mind'. They acquired a warrant for his apprehension.

It would be almost a decade before the warrant came to fruition. McKinsey decamped, changed his name and determinedly 'kept out of the way'. His medicines remained on sale via a Truro chemist, but the Baron himself commenced 'dodging about all over England', always remaining just out of Captain Bent's reach.

At last, in 1884, he was arrested at Twickenham under the alias of Alfred Norrish, saying: 'I know I'm the man; it's no good denying it. I was a fool to let them "cop" so many of the pamphlets; I ought to have destroyed them.'

After nine years on the run, Henry McKinsey was tried at Exeter and acquitted. His Life-Preserving Katapotia survived well into the twentieth century, remaining 'the most scientifically prepared medicines ever compounded by human skill'.

11

A SOURCE OF CONSIDERABLE TROUBLE

'I can cure you,' the representative of the Ladies' Medical Association told 37-year-old Julia Ann Ralph. 'If you will trust in me and the Lord, take a few drops from this bottle, and pay me half a guinea down and undertake to pay half a guinea in six weeks' time, then you will soon be a different woman.'

It was 1892 and Julia was dying of cancer. The doctors had told her there was nothing more they could do. Her six children, the youngest only a year old, must prepare to say goodbye to their mother. So when Maria Owen came to the door, explaining that she was a cancer specialist sent by a worried neighbour, George Ralph directed her to his wife's bedroom.

Maria Owen measured out the drops of her elixir, collected the 10s 6d from Mr Ralph, spent a few moments sympathising with the children and left. That was the last they saw of her. There was no such thing as The Ladies' Medical Association, the elixir was a solution of vinegar and soap in water and Owen was a career fraudster for whom building the hopes of dying people was just a means to her own survival.

On this occasion, she was locked up for a year. By the time she got out, the grim reaper had done an excellent job of relieving Julia Ralph's pain forever.

The 'bogus lady doctor', described in 1890 when she was 41 as 'a woman of strong build […] attired in a broad-brimmed hat, which was jauntily placed on one side of her head', became so familiar to the courts that newspaper reports of her trials seem almost weary in tone.

The people targeted by Maria Owen were impoverished and probably lacking education, but their responses to her attempts at fraud reveal them not as a mass of credulous idiots but as human individuals made vulnerable by disease, poverty and worry. And when Owen failed to defraud them – which she often did – it was the patients and their relatives who can take the credit for bringing her to justice.

Born Maria Gwyn in Ross-on-Wye, she started her criminal career in around 1886 in partnership with her husband, Frederick Owen (or Owens), a dentist and herbalist who posed as a qualified physician under a variety of names. Maria had several convictions during that year for drunkenness, larceny and obtaining alms by false pretences, but then she and Frederick devised a more complex scheme to dupe servant girls by telling their fortunes. When the Owens informed a customer called Mrs Davies that her husband was having it off with a dark-eyed girl and had got her pregnant, but that the philanderer would be killed and Mrs Davies would marry a rich man, they got caught out. Mrs Davies had been sent as a decoy by her husband, the local bobby, and the pair spent a month in gaol.

In 1887, Frederick Owen attempted to hang himself and may subsequently have undergone his first sojourn in an asylum, but within less than a year he was back to convincing people he was qualified as a doctor. At the Hereford Quarter Sessions in summer 1888, he was indicted on four counts of obtaining money and goods (namely bacon) by false pretences and stealing a pair of woollen stockings. His methods of gaining patients' confidence included telling them he was an agent for Warner's Safe Cure, a popular patent medicine. He might also say he had been sent by a respected person such as the vicar's wife, or claim to be the nephew of a genuine local practitioner who happened to be called Dr Owen. These ploys worked on a client named Mary Bruton, who parted with 10s for medicine only to feel less convinced when he returned to her house pissed as a fart and saying he'd turned his wife into a cat.

Neither her husband's arrest, nor her feline state, put Maria Owen off trying to con 18-year-old Wilson Russell out of £1 for medicine for his sick mother. Russell intended to get the money from his employer but had second thoughts and went to the police station, discovering there that Owen had just been arrested for something else. So while her husband was being sentenced to five years' penal servitude, Owen got her own prison term of six months. Once out, she immediately carried on as a sole operator in the business of scamming the public.

A consistent modus operandi emerges from reports of Owen's convictions. She appears to have prepared her attempts by scouting the neighbourhood for ill people and picking up on gossip about their condition. She sussed out the names of the mark's friends or other trusted acquaintances and tailored her story to the individual. In the case of Julia Ralph, Owen said she had been asked to attend by Mrs Clarke, a neighbour and friend who was worried about Mrs Ralph's condition. Wilson Russell's mother had been an inpatient at Worcester Infirmary, so Owen claimed that one of the doctors there had sent her. To deflect any awkward questions at the hospital, she told her patients not to let the staff there know about her price for the medicine, as she would get into trouble for selling it so cheaply. Although she sometimes managed to afford lodgings, there were other times when she was of no fixed address and in one case in the depths of winter 1889, she played on the compassion of a Stourbridge couple who allowed her to stay the night and gave her money for her railway fair the next morning.

Even if someone wasn't ill, however, Owen would try her luck at convincing them they were. In Aston in 1890, she persuaded a woman to part with what was literally her last shilling by terrifying her with a diagnosis of terminal heart disease. Another woman, whose nose had been disfigured by cancer, paid 4s 6d on Owen's promise that 'If I don't put a new nose on your face in six weeks' time I'll refund the money.' Neither nose nor refund ever materialised.

If it weren't for the immorality of preying on disadvantaged people for whom death was an ever-lurking threat, Owen's determination and persistence would be rather admirable. Even when a mark was uninterested or sceptical, she did not give up until all ways of extracting cash, goods, or at best a bed for the night, had failed.

When she tried her heart disease trick on Mrs Cooper of Aston, her potential victim tried to put her off by saying she had no money, so Owen insisted on writing to Mrs Cooper's husband at work.

Will Mr Cooper approve for his wife to come under our treatment, as I am sure I can cure her, as she is sinking fast; in fact, I would not take her in hand after today. Your wife will have medicine 3 months 5s. down 5s. 6d. month. The pills and medicine she is now taking you will find do her no good.

Signed, EMILY PEARCE, the Hospital.

When Mr Cooper arrived home, he regarded his wife's visitor with suspicion and tried to discover more about her role at the hospital. Her reply was that she dressed all the bad legs. Cunningly, Mr Cooper suggested that he have a think about the medicine and meet her at the hospital to discuss it later that evening, but Owen was ready with an excuse about having to sit up all night with another patient. At this point, it might have been advisable for Owen to cut her losses and run for it, but she persevered with her plan, asking Mr Cooper to go and borrow half a crown from friends. Unfortunately for her, the 'friend' accompanying his return was Detective Joseph Whitcroft of the Aston police force.

While Owen sometimes presented herself as a nurse, she also adopted the title of 'doctress' or 'lady doctor', presenting 'such a polite form' as to be convincing in this role. At a time when there were only around 100 female doctors practising in England and Wales, perhaps the element of mystique surrounding Owen's supposed occupation further discombobulated her victims. Her polite demeanour, however, tended to wear off rapidly at the moment of arrest.

In the police lock-up, awaiting her hearing in the Cooper case, Owen was 'a source of considerable trouble'. First she claimed to be dying of heart disease. When no one believed her, she said she was pregnant. No one believed that, either, and the only labour in her near future was hard labour in prison.

Frederick Owen's release from penal servitude in 1893 did not lead to a happy-ever-after moment for him and Maria. He was removed to Hampshire County Asylum and spent the remainder of his life – more than thirty years – between there and the equivalent institution in Dorchester.

Maria Owen got into trouble at least once more, when she was arrested on the Great Western Railway platform at Neath, claiming to have been sent by God to cure fits, but after 1895 she faded into obscurity. In spite of her crimes, it is difficult not to feel some sympathy for this chancer of no fixed abode, who 'seemed very wet and tired' when she begged a night's lodging of the couple in Stourbridge. Her persistence in the face of suspicion, conviction and hard labour hint at desperation and a desire to get any roof – even a prison one – over her head.

She might never have been proprietor of a famous patent medicine, placed expensive advertisements in the newspapers, or driven in a flashy carriage, but her career gives a glimpse of medical fraud's potential in the criminal underworld.

12

YOU WILL BECOME LIKE THE DAINTY GIRL

How was a patent medicine proprietor to market a cure for plumpness? The anguish of suffering a terminal disease, the embarrassment of having picked up more than you bargained for in the extra-marital bed, or the disgust of entertaining an intestinal parasite could lead to a desperate search for remedies. But being a few pounds heavier than the next person was hardly life-threatening. How could a weight loss medicine become a commercial success?

That was the challenge faced by the maker of Figuroids in 1907. Other companies were already recognising the potential of fat-reducing products. The new U.S. brand Marmola was manipulating the self-perception of women with a cleverly low-key introduction to the market and the Antipon Company was bottling a solution of citric acid and claiming that it would remove 'a considerable quantity of the most unhealthy fat' within twenty-four hours.

Commercial weight-loss products were not new. For decades, Allan's Anti-Fat, containing an extract of the seaweed species *Fucus vesiculosis* (bladderwrack), had been the 'celebrated remedy for corpulency'. Its advertisements in 1879 asked readers to picture the scene:

> An exceedingly fat lady puffing like a steam engine, and clinging
> to the arm of a small wiry gentleman, whose face has become very
> red either from the unusual exercise or from the consciousness that a
> hundred eyes are looking at him with a ha! ha! in each pupil.

Obesity, according to Allan's Anti-Fat, was a source of shame. The obese woman should recognise herself as an embarrassment and a caricature; the male reader should look at his wife and wonder whether he became an emasculated source of general amusement when seen in her company. Nearly thirty years later, a Marmola advertisement, disguised as a news snippet in the *London Daily Mail*, went even further to ensure its potential customers were sufficiently unhappy with their bodies:

IS FATNESS A SOCIAL OFFENCE?

'The female form, being capable of expressing a supreme degree of grace, should be an inspiration to our daily lives and lead up to higher ideals of beauty,' said an art lecturer lately. Therefore the fat woman is an enemy to the artistic uplift, for she is entirely too heavy for any wings of fancy to raise.

Marmola's advertising presented the product as just one ingredient in a homespun weight-loss recipe that could be made up by any pharmacist. The product was more dangerous than many of its harmless and ineffective contemporaries as it contained desiccated thyroid material that might have caused some weight loss but also had a risk of side effects.

George Dixon, managing director of the Figuroid Company, initially took a different marketing tack. Rather than laughing at his audience or insulting them, he flattered their reason and common sense. The unique selling point of Figuroids was that they were scientific – indeed they had been 'DISCOVERED THROUGH AN ACCIDENT, while making Scientific

Investigations in the Laboratory' – and their rivals' advertising was born of ignorance.

Dixon was already successful in the patent medicine business. A qualified doctor from Brockville, Ontario, he had come to England in the mid-1890s and begun promoting Dr Campbell's Red Blood Forming Capsuloids, a haemoglobin preparation to treat anaemia. With a new century approaching, the old-fashioned name was dropped and the product became Capsuloids, making £497 17s 6d in 1899. It was joined by other remedies, including Cicfa for indigestion and by 1908 Dixon's businesses were making an average yearly profit of £10,500.

Although Capsuloids weren't promoted heavily until 1899, their early newspaper adverts employed an interesting marketing technique – making the reader feel unwell enough to need the product. A diagram of the heart accompanied a case study that probably did induce a certain pallor in the complexions of its readers:

> He drank fresh blood every day at the Butcher's. His doctor had ordered him to do so. He was Pale, Anaemic, had Indigestion, Constipation, Bloating, Palpitation, and a cough, and was spitting up considerable, and he had lost over 21lbs. He grew sick of the smell and taste of Fresh Blood and could not swallow it any longer.

The doctor then advised the patient to try Capsuloids, which makes one wonder why he put the poor fellow through all that palaver in the first place.

Visiting Denmark in 1899, Dixon was in the Tivoli Gardens when he noticed a young woman in charge of a lottery wheel. He offered Jeanne Amalie Hansen, then 20 years old, a role translating English Capsuloid advertisements into Danish. She subsequently became manager of the company's new Copenhagen branch and the possessor of a comfortable bed, which accommodated Dixon whenever he was in Denmark on business over the next five years.

Their intimacy, and the fact that Dixon wrote to her saying, 'If I were well, little girl, would you marry me?' led Miss Hansen to believe, not unreasonably, that he wanted to marry her. As his visits to Denmark became less frequent, Miss Hansen travelled to London for answers, only to be confused by her lover's shifty behaviour and lack of affection. It was only after returning to Copenhagen that she read in the *Smart Set* paper of Dixon's marriage to Marie Bokenham, a gentleman's daughter whom he had known only two months. Miss Hansen sued him for breach of promise.

Although Dixon denied proposing to Miss Hansen, he told the court that if he had, it was before he knew she was unchaste. She had been seduced by a German baron at the age of 17, but according to her, Dixon had known about this from the beginning and wasn't half as bothered by it when he was trying to get his end away. Miss Hansen was awarded £1,500 damages – the best part of Dixon's personal annual income at that time.

Dixon was getting familiar with the High Court of Justice – a month before the breach of promise case, he was there to appeal against the registrar's decision to reject his trademark application for Tablones, an indigestion remedy. Burroughs, Wellcome & Co. opposed the application, offering evidence of the public confusing the product with their own famous Tabloids. The judge rejected Dixon's appeal.

With the Denmark branch of the Capsuloid Company wound up in the face of a savaging from the Danish newspapers and Tablones down on their luck, Dixon began a new venture – The Figuroid Company, established in November 1907. The product, a 'Gentle, Scientific, Natural and Absolutely Safe Obesity Cure', claimed to start a scientific process in the body that would allow the consumer to breathe, sweat, wee and poo their fat away. 'This leaflet is for those who think and reason

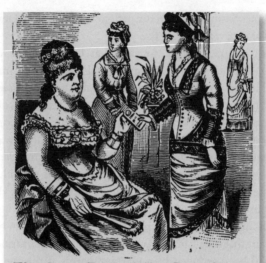

The Great Remedy for Corpulence

ALLAN'S ANTI-FAT

is composed of purely vegetable ingredients, and is perfectly harmless. It acts upon the food in the stomach, preventing its being converted into fat. Taken in accordance with directions, **it will reduce a fat person from two to five pounds per week.**

"Corpulence is not only a disease itself, but the harbinger of others." So wrote Hippocrates two thousand years ago, and what was true then is none the less so to-day.

Before using the Anti-Fat, make a careful note of your weight, and after one week's treatment note the improvement, not only in diminution of weight, but in the improved appearance and vigorous and healthy feeling it imparts to the patient. It is an unsurpassed blood-purifier and has been found especially efficacious in curing Rheumatism.

CERTIFICATE.—I have subjected Allan's Anti-Fat to chemical analysis, examined the process of its manufacture, and can truly say that the ingredients of which it is composed are entirely vegetable, and cannot but act favorably upon the system, and is well calculated to attain the object for which it is intended.   W. B. DRAKE, *Analytical Chemist.*

Allan's Anti-Fat. *US National Library of Medicine*

and use their common sense,' proclaimed an advertising pamphlet in *The Girl's Own Paper* in December 1907. Other anti-fat remedies, the pamphlet said, would promise to shrink fat within the body or somehow render it non-existent. Only those who 'do not use their common sense' would believe this. As Figuroids' readers would understand, no weight loss could occur unless fat was removed from the body altogether – and this could only happen if it were transferred from the adipose cells to the capillaries and there oxidised for excretion. Exactly how Figuroids did this wasn't clear, but the pamphlet would equip the reader to 'explain it all scientifically to your friends'. Before, during and after diagrams illustrated how the fat cells would shrink once Figuroids had done their work. The fat:

> must first be caused to pass out of the adipose cells into the little blood vessels, and it must there be oxidised and so converted into carbon-dioxide and water vapour, both of which are then eliminated readily from the body through the four great eliminating channels, the lungs, skin, kidneys and bowels.

Underlying the scientific veneer, however, was a subtle appeal to the reader to feel disgust at her own body. The pamphlet's focus on science did not allow for comment on art and aesthetics, but the unhealthy biological processes endured by the overweight person gave scope for inducing self-loathing.

In Figuroids' 'scientific' view of the fat person, sweaty, red and shiny skin formed the unattractive exterior to a body full of acidic blood, its water content forced out of constricted capillaries. Gout and rheumatism lurked around the joints, dilated fat cells blocked the circulation and palpitations pounded through the heart's coating of fat. The reader was asked repeatedly to 'look again at the diagrams' and picture what was lurking under her skin.

And the company seemed fairly confident that it would be a 'her'. The illustration used on both Figuroids' magazine inserts and its newspaper adverts showed three figures side by side – the same woman in her 'stout', 'medium' and 'dainty' incarnations. Although the copy did not rule out male customers, referring to the distribution of fat in male bodies too, the aspirational shrinkage in the illustration showed women the ideal to which they should strive. 'IF you are like the STOUT girl – you will become like the MEDIUM girl – and finally like the DAINTY girl – by taking Figuroids.'

In 1908, the focus on science slipped. French women visiting the Franco-British Exhibition were sporting a new fashion – the sheath dress. The opportunity was too good and the Figuroids Company could not resist invoking their elegant image to convince portly Brits to shape up. An unillustrated advert began, in the Marmola style, as a news story. The headline asked:

CAN STOUT WOMEN WEAR THE SHEATH GOWN?

A fat person can only wear what suits her own figure, and frequently suspects that her unfashionable attire and awkward personal appearance are the cause of much of the tittering she happens to overhear. This is a distressing condition for a woman to have to endure. The lithe, vivacious movements of her friend, attired in the latest fashionable gown, make her more and more desirous, like Hamlet, 'that this too, too solid flesh would melt, thaw and resolve itself into a dew.'

The reader, whether really overweight or not, is prompted to hear any laughter as directed at her. Maybe her body is not good enough. Maybe her clothes look awful. Even her personality is suspect – she lacks the vivacity of her friend. The only accepted response is to long to melt away – perhaps, like Hamlet, wishing that her entire existence would disappear. The answer to the headline was, of course, yes, provided the stout women used Figuroids to slim down first.

Figuroids were attractively presented. Each tablet bore the product name and was wrapped in silver paper, but the product within was useless. An analysis by the BMA in 1908 revealed that they comprised bicarbonate of soda, tartaric acid, sodium chloride, phenolphthalein, hexamethyline-tetramine, talc and gum – none of which had any application for obesity.

Figuroids might have been promoted through a lens of science and rationality, but they were ineffective. And underneath the attractive exterior lurked the perennially successful advertising message – you are not good enough.

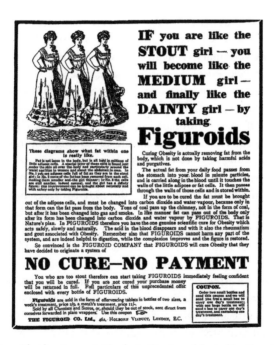

Figuroids advertisement. *Manchester Courier and Lancashire General Advertiser, Tuesday 17 March 1908. Image © Northcliffe Media Limited. Image created courtesy of THE BRITISH LIBRARY BOARD. Image reproduced with kind permission of the British Newspaper Archive (www.britishnewspaperarchive.co.uk)*

13

WHEN EXHAUSTED HE WILL BEAR IT IN MIND

There was never any shortage of people wanting to be singers.

Dr Robert Carter Moffat, Professor of Chemistry at Glasgow Veterinary College, was one of them. His own vocal chords, producers of 'a poor, miserable, squeaky affair', became the guinea pig for more than thirty years of study, obsession, travel and experimentation. The result of his efforts was an invention that transformed his warblings into 'a pure tenor of extraordinary range' and hit the advertising columns as the next big thing in voice cultivation.

But when an improved version of his 'Ammoniaphone' received a British patent in 1884, Dr Moffat's name was nowhere on the papers. In his place as 'inventor' was Cornelius Bennett Harness, an unqualified medical electrician whose fortune was founded on one simple motto: 'Sell goods'.

What was the Ammoniaphone? Elegant and flute-like, the device consisted of a slender pewter instrument about 25 inches long. Unlike a flute, however, it sported a mouthpiece in the centre and a valve at either end. Within was an absorbent material saturated with ingredients that Dr Moffat claimed would artificially 'Italianize' British air, bringing the abilities of the great Italian singers nearer to the ordinary person's grasp. All the aspiring singer had to do was place their lips over the central knob and suck.

Such unusual claims attracted amused attention from the press and in January 1884 the Occasional Notes section of the *Pall Mall Gazette* carried a paragraph about the invention. The Ammoniaphone, it reported, had been tested on Scottish choirs with extraordinary results and was sure to be in demand in England, where the opera companies could certainly do with improvement.

It was just a quirky space-filler, but the novelty and improbability of the Ammoniaphone caught the eye of other newsmen and reprints of the article multiplied across the globe. Within a few weeks, the *Pall Mall Gazette*'s postbag bulged with letters asking for the inventor's address. It was an opportunity too good for the *Gazette*'s innovative editor, W.T. Stead, to pass up, and the paper sent a 'sceptical representative' to interview Dr Moffat. At a time when press interviews themselves were something new and different, the insight it gave into the Ammoniaphone's history and the character of its inventor was the best advertisement the product could have had.

Moffat was staying at 205 Regent Street, then the headquarters of C.B. Harness's Medical Battery Company (and next door to the premises later inhabited by A.L. Pointing's Antidipso and Thermal Bath companies). According to the interview, the 'tall, slenderly built Scotchman' (who was then 42 years old) met his visitor's questions courteously, even when they did not take the matter very seriously: 'Is there any possibility of your transforming my voice into that of a Mr Sims Reeves by a few whiffs of what I may call your condensed essence of Italian air?' Dr Moffat then related the tale of three decades of dedication to voice improvement.

At the age of just 12, Moffat 'conceived the rather curious idea that the beauty of Italian tone was due to something in the air of Italy not found elsewhere'. He began conducting experiments – not detailed in the interview – and continued these through his studies at the Royal College of Surgeons

Edinburgh and after his appointment as Professor of Chemistry and Technological Lecturer at Glasgow in his twenties. As a chemical analyst, Moffat combined his academic role with corporate assignments, and it was one of these that took him to Italy in 1874, leading to a breakthrough in his hitherto futile investigations.

Moffat was there for five weeks to examine the commercial viability of extracting bitumen from the limestone, but no sooner did he set foot in Pescara than he was aware of a phenomenon linked to his lifelong obsession. The 'peculiar yellow-green tint of the vegetation and the sombre autumnal appearance of all nature' formed a sharp contrast to the Glasgow summer he had left behind. Moffat's chemical knowledge told him there must be something special in the air.

In the spare time between his tasks for the mineral oil company, Moffat analysed the dewdrops and discovered the presence of hydrogen peroxide and free ammonia. Going 'from valley to valley and plain to plain', he conducted a further seventy-two analyses of the dew and air with the same result. The chemicals were present in particularly large quantities in the region where the great tenor, Antonio Giuglini – conveniently well-known in London – had been born. Not only that, but visits to the local peasants' huts revealed that 'the men in particular could produce those high, open, tenor notes'.

For Moffat, this was sufficient evidence that the 'curious idea' of his boyhood really was true. Back at home, he resigned all of his academic and corporate posts and retired to a Lanarkshire farm to set up his own laboratory, working night and day at perfecting a way to make practical use of his discovery. It took him nine and a half years, but at last the Ammoniaphone was ready. Dr Moffat had changed his own voice from 'the worst example of a thin, weak drawing-roon tenor' to one that the *Pall Mall Gazette*'s representative witnessed first hand as 'full of massive power and singularly rich'. The journalist had a go of

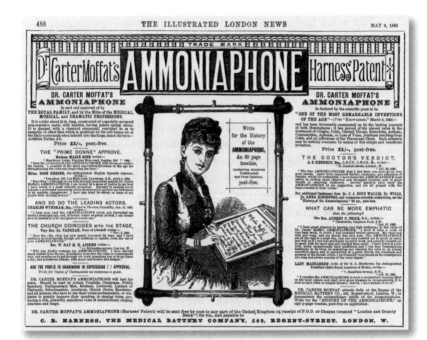

Ammoniaphone. *Author's collection*

the Ammoniaphone too and had to admit that his vocal range
had increased by three notes.

The *Pall Mall Gazette* interview ended with a variation on
the joke from the original news snippet that had inspired it:

In a short time, therefore, we may expect to hear the whole population
of London warbling like Italian prime donne, but before that blessed
consummation is reached it is proposed to raise a public subscription
to present an Ammoniaphone to several well-known members of
Parliament and not a few pulpit orators, whose voices at present are
terribly in need of an Italian tone.

The story had everything the Ammoniaphone's promoters could have hoped for. A romantic Italian setting, a hero's alchemical quest to discover the truth, the conversion of the sceptic and the resulting invention's potential to change the reader's own life.

On the day that the interview appeared in the *Pall Mall Gazette*, a patent was issued to Cornelius Bennett Harness for an 'Apparatus for facilitating the inhalation of medicated vapours'. Perhaps Moffat had exaggerated the extent of his commitment to the Ammoniaphone, for he had sold the patent rights to Harness for £2,000 worth of Medical Battery Company shares.

The company, initially a subsidiary of Harness's Pall Mall Electrical Association, mainly sold electropathic belts, devices that capitalised on the widespread interest in the potential of electricity. Electric belts had been a staple of the less reputable sections of the medical fringe for decades, the mystique of electricity providing a cover for the provision of fraudulent products. Harness had received a patent for his version in 1883, allegedly having appropriated the invention of one George Baker, whose family ended up in poverty while Harness was at the height of his success. Dr Moffat was more fortunate in the short term as his knowledge of and enthusiasm for the Ammoniaphone, plus his lecturing ability, were too useful for Harness to dismiss. Moffat remained with the Medical Battery Company to promote the instrument through public demonstrations and it was still known as 'Dr Carter Moffat's Ammoniaphone'. By 1886 the voice improvement aspect of the Ammoniaphone was joined by claims that it could cure lung conditions including asthma and tuberculosis.

Advertising via newspapers and pamphlets was handled by Harness and his copywriters. Its associations with talent and fame made the Ammoniaphone perfect for a form of marketing not always easily obtainable for other products – the celebrity testimonial. Along with the numerous ordinary joes who wrote in saying the Ammoniaphone was 'magical' and 'wonderful', adverts featured the names of famous performers, including Madame Marie Rose, Madame Rose Hersee and Lillie Langtry.

Harness's method of gathering these testimonials was not the height of scrupulousness, for any high-profile person with an Ammoniaphone in their possession was fair game for ending up in an advert. Harness only had to make sure they owned an Ammoniaphone by sending them a free one and then writing to them periodically offering to replenish the chemicals inside it. Even the most non-committal of replies could then be manipulated into an endorsement. Italian opera singer Adelina Patti, 'the peerless "Queen of Song"' was reasonably enthusiastic: 'I have used the Ammoniaphone and found its effects most beneficial,' but other correspondents probably did not realise they were giving testimonials. Lady Sophia MacNamara, lady-in-waiting to Princess Louise, wrote to thank Harness for the offer to recharge the royal inhalers. She would 'certainly inform him when the Ammoniaphones want replenishing; at present they are in good order'. Although she gave no opinion on the instruments' efficacy or even any indication that they had ever been used, her letter was enough to get her name and prestigious Kensington Palace address into the Ammoniaphone adverts in 1885.

Prime Minister W.E. Gladstone was even less effusive – his secretary H.W. Primrose informed Harness, 'Mr Gladstone has received your letter of the 9th, and desires me to thank you for your kind offer to recharge his Ammoniaphone. When exhausted he will bear it in mind.' Strongly implying that Gladstone did not actually use the instrument, the note nevertheless qualified as a testimonial for Harness's purposes

THROAT & CHEST COMPLAINTS

May be immediately relieved by a few inhalations through

Dr. Carter Moffat's world-famed Ammoniaphone.

THE
AMMONIAPHONE
CURES ASTHMA.

AMMONIAPHONE
CURES BRONCHITIS.

AMMONIAPHONE
CURES CATARRH.

AMMONIAPHONE
FOR THE VOICE.

AMMONIAPHONE
ADVICE FREE.

AMMONIAPHONE
PAMPHLET FREE.

Read what the Clergy say:—

"Conscientiously testify to its value."—*Rev. A. C. Price, Clapham Park, S.W.*

"It strengthens the voice."—*Rev. C. J. Salisbury, Newport.*

"It is a wonderful invention."—*Rev. S. E. Nichols, Wimborne, Minster.*

"Has done me good service."—*Rev. E. Singleton, Spalding.*

"It is worthy of all confidence."—*Rev. John Mitchell, Edinburgh.*

SPEEDILY CURES

ASTHMA, BRONCHITIS, & SORE THROAT.

It also Strengthens and Enriches the Voice, and is Invaluable to Public Speakers, Vocalists, Clergymen, &c.

IMMEDIATE RELIEF GUARANTEED

Used and Recommended by Thousands, including H.R.H. THE PRINCESS OF WALES, Right Hon. W. E. GLADSTONE, Madame ADELINA PATTI, Mrs. LANGTRY, and the principal Doctors and Clergymen throughout the country.

ADVICE AND PAMPHLET POST-FREE.

Dr. CARTER MOFFAT'S AMMONIAPHONE will be sent free by post to any part of the United Kingdom on receipt of P.O.O. or Cheque for 21s., and payable to

MEDICAL BATTERY CO., LIMITED,
52, OXFORD STREET, LONDON, W. (Corner of Rathbone Place.)

ADVICE TO INVALIDS

Before you waste your time and money on nauseous drugs and quack medicines, Mr. C. B. HARNESS (*President of the British Association of Medical Electricians*) recommends you to pay a visit to the Electropathic and Zander Institute, 52, Oxford Street, London, W. (corner of Rathbone Place), where, by means of experiments and testimonials, he will be able to prove to you conclusively that his world-famed electropathic Battery Belt is certain to cure, and has cured, the most obstinate cases of nervous exhaustion, physical debility, hypochondriasis, melancholia, or any sign of premature decline of vital energy consequent upon overstrain. Harness' electropathic treatment needs only to be more widely known to be universally adopted, and it is for this reason that we are now advertising so largely. The surest proof we have of the success of our treatment is that almost every patient who has adopted it has introduced several other sufferers. Harness' electropathic Belt has also relieved and cured hundreds of men and women suffering from rheumatic affections, indigestion, constipation, liver and kidney diseases, etc., and is the most natural and certain means of obtaining health strength, and vital energy. Pamphlet and advice free of charge. Residents at a distance, and those unable to call at 52, Oxford Street, London, W., should write at once for private advice form. Advice free, personally or by letter. Note the address carefully, lest you forget it, and call or write at once to Mr. C. B. HARNESS, Consulting Medical Electrician, The Medical Battery Company, Limited, 52, Oxford Street, London, W. (corner of Rathbone Place). All communications treated as strictly private.

RUPTURE SUCCESSFULLY TREATED.

Sufferers may save themselves a lifetime of discomfort and torture by being properly fitted with Mr. C. B. Harness' new perfect appliance. Examinations free by a most experienced and skilful surgeon at the Medical Battery Company's Electropathic and Zander Institute, 52, Oxford Street, London, W. (corner of Rathbone Place). Note only address, and call to-day if possible. Send for Pamphlet and copies of Testimonials.

Ammoniaphone. *Author's collection*

and from then on the company lost no opportunity to link the premier's name with the Ammoniaphone.

Given that Prime Ministers rarely enjoy universal popularity, this ploy sometimes backfired. Speaking at a concert organised by Colonel J.H. Mapleton (a famous music agent and theatre owner, who had been the late Giuglini's manager), Dr Moffat's mention of Gladstone provoked 'a storm of hisses'.

Other concerts, however, proved a successful way of getting the Ammoniaphone in front of an appreciative audience. Singers genuinely keen to support the invention would perform 'before and after' songs and Dr Moffat would point out the 'fuller and richer effect' of the voice. Having been invited to an enjoyable – and free – concert, no one was churlish enough to disagree.

The Medical Battery Company's opulent new premises at 52 Oxford Street housed an Ammoniaphone exhibition room, allowing potential purchasers to try it out in surroundings of which only a superior product could be worthy. Adverts described it as:

> The spacious musical saloon, furnished in the most recherché manner with a magnificent Chickering concert grand piano and a powerful American organ, is daily frequented by the elite of the haut ton and of the medical, musical and dramatic professions.

The Ammoniaphone enjoyed almost ten years of popularity, but in the end it was dragged down by the less savoury side of Harness's business. In 1893, the paper that had helped shoot the instrument to fame, the *Pall Mall Gazette*, assisted its demise with a series of articles condemning Harness as 'a man of no pretensions whatever to scientific or medical knowledge, but a common, illiterate and unscrupulous charlatan'.

The *Electrical Review* had already printed an exposé of Harness's activities and he had also had a run-in with the

British Medical Journal, but the *Gazette* brought the issues to a wider audience. The focus of the 'Harness "Electropathic" Swindle' series was the company's other products – its electric belts and magnetic corsets – rather than the Ammoniaphone, but the whole venture suffered, proving to Harness that some publicity could, after all, be bad publicity.

The *Pall Mall Gazette* presented Harness's customers as poor, uneducated victims preyed upon by a fraudster as ignorant of electricity as he was of the Queen's English. The electric belts did not work and people were being 'drawn to that mysterious word "electricity" like moths to a candle'. Although this was not very flattering to the intelligence of Harness's customers, many wrote in to describe their experiences and thank the *Gazette* for publishing the articles.

Swamped with demands for refunds, Harness resigned as managing director. But that was no escape from his tribulations. In November 1893, just a few weeks after the *Gazette* began its series, he and a business associate, Dr James McCully (originally a qualified physician but struck off the Medical Register), were arrested and charged with unlawfully conspiring to defraud. One report of the case said that Harness had been questioned about his medical expertise. He'd been asked: 'Do you know anything about pathology? Do you know what pathology means?' He replied: 'The study of medicine, I suppose.'

His apparent ignorance had been a feature of the *Pall Mall Gazette*'s article, which quoted J. Jerritt, a former employee of the Medical Battery Company. At his job interview for the post of lecturer in electro-physiology, Jerritt remembered Harness saying: 'My electrical knowledge may be put into a nutshell. I believe in attending to the commercial part, and selling the goods.'

Dr McCully was found not guilty but the jury couldn't agree about Harness. The courts ordered that the company be wound up. Almost immediately in 1894 Harness tried to resurrect it as the Medical Electrical Institute and was allowed to do so on condition that it was under control of a qualified medic. The creditors and shareholders of the old company unanimously agreed that it should go ahead, and Mr Harness became manager of the new company on a salary of £600 a year. The public, however, were now wise to him, and he went bust within a few months.

The Ammoniaphone disappeared along with Harness's electropathic belts and electric corsets, but at least for a time it had captured the public's imagination and provided inspiration – literally – to the most unprepossessing of drawing-room warblers.

14

THOU CHURCH-YARD PIMP

What is any quack worth his or her salt to do in the face of criticism? The answer in 1804 was exactly the same as it is now – turn nasty and threaten to sue the arse off everyone. When Ching's Worm Lozenges were responsible for the death of a toddler, their proprietor saw fit to make the family's life even more of a misery.

The contents of the Worm Lozenges were not completely secret, for unlike many patent remedies, they were actually patented. John Ching had filed a specification in 1796 detailing his method of making them. His decision to render the ingredients in what the *Medical Observer* termed 'humble dog Latin' came under criticism as an attempt to obscure the recipe, but it was clear that the lozenges contained nothing original in the way of anthelmintics.

There were two kinds of lozenge – yellow and brown – to be taken at different times of day. The yellow contained English saffron and the brown contained jalap, but they shared their main ingredients – sugar and white panacea of mercury. This preparation of calomel (mercurous chloride) washed in spirits of wine was out of fashion with most doctors and chemists, who did not view it as any more efficacious than calomel alone and had 'expunged the ridiculous title from their pharmacopoeias'.

The average punter, however, could not be expected to make investigations at the patent office every time they wanted to buy something. The patent might have revealed the contents of the lozenges, but the marketing didn't. After John Ching's death in around 1800, the medicine ostensibly remained under the proprietorship of his widow Rebecca, who held the patent, but it was advertised and distributed by Ching's business partner, Richard Butler of No. 4 Cheapside. Butler's travelling sales agents were under strict instructions to assure customers that the lozenges contained 'not a single particle' of mercury. Even if asked outright, the travellers were expected to deny the poison's presence and emphasise the lozenges' safety.

On 4 December 1803, a little boy called Thomas Clayton, aged 3, was given the lozenges, followed three days later by a repeat dose. He went into a high state of salivation – one of the symptoms of mercury poisoning. His parents sent for medical help, but to no avail:

> ... the mouth ulcerated, the Teeth dropped out, the Hands contracted, and a Complaint was made, of a pricking Pain in them and the Feet, the Body became flushed and spotted, and at last Black, Convulsions succeeded, attended with a slight delirium; and a Mortification destroyed the Face, which proceeding to the Brain, put a period (after indescribable Torments) to the life of the little sufferer, on Sunday, the 1st instant, Twenty-Eight Days after he had taken the Poisonous Lozenges.

The coroner's verdict was 'Poisoned by Ching's Worm Lozenges' and the details of the case appeared as a warning to parents on a handbill written by the child's father, also called Thomas Clayton. Clayton's business as a printer and bookseller put him in a good position to publicise the tragedy by personally delivering leaflets all around his local neighbourhood in Kingston-upon-Hull. In them, he noted that the main Hull papers (the *Packet* and the *Advertiser*) had ignored both the death and the coroner's verdict – probably because they received so much advertising revenue from Ching and Butler.

Signing himself R. Ching, Butler responded with a broadside of his own, attacking the grieving father and threatening to prosecute him for publishing the case. Butler asserted that he 'cannot calmly surrender the unsullied Reputation, which, for a period of ten years, has distinguished the most invaluable Vermifuge that has ever fallen to the lot of man to discover'.

The cause of death, he said, must have been one of the Worm Lozenges' inferior imitators, and Clayton's accusations were nothing but 'malicious invective', 'AN INFAMOUS ASSERTION and ABOMINABLE FALSEHOOD', which 'FLAGRANTLY LIBELLED TRUTH'. These handbills were printed by Robert Peck of the *Hull Packet* – who, like many newspaper printers, was a local stockist of patent remedies and was not about to jeopardise this source of income.

Perhaps Clayton's grief and campaigning activities led him to neglect his business, or perhaps he was already in financial trouble, but he was declared bankrupt about a month after his son's death. Although the newspapers had not reported the poisoning, they were quick to advertise the sale of all the Claytons' property. In a particularly despicable act, Robert Peck allegedly turned up at the sale and boasted to Mrs Clayton that her husband would be severely punished for the libel. Thomas Clayton attributed his wife's subsequent miscarriage to the distress Peck had caused her.

Clayton wanted to take the precaution of getting a written copy of the coroner's verdict, but when he went to pick it up, he discovered that the coroner 'had not time' to do it. The Deputy Town Clerk was equally unhelpful and although an acquaintance advised Clayton to apply to the Assizes judges, Clayton was unsure how to go about this. Fortunately, Butler was all talk and did not proceed with the prosecution.

By 1805 Clayton had managed to get back in business as a printer and published *An Essay on Quackery, and the dreadful consequences arising from taking advertised medicines; with remarks on their Fatal Effects, with an account of a recent death occasioned by a Quack medicine.* The anonymous publication was sometimes attributed to Thomas Clayton himself, but a letter to the *Medical Observer* in 1806 implies that it was compiled by his brother, M.J. Clayton. The 140-page book is emotional, condemning the 'miscreants who have been too long thriving by the destruction of their credulous fellow creatures' as 'more deserving of condign punishment, than the vilest assassin that ever suffered for his villainy, at the gallows, or on the wheel' and characterising Butler in poetry as:

Base, sordid monster! mercenary slave!
Thou Church-yard Pimp and Pander to the Grave

Much of it comprises reproduced excerpts from other writers and reviews were far from glowing. The *Anti-Jacobin Review*, though sympathising with the author's intentions, criticised the book as 'made up of scraps in prose and verse, collected from every quarter and put together without attention to arrangement', while the *British Critic and Quarterly Theological Review* labelled it a 'farrago'.

The author, however, was his own worst critic, describing his book in the *Medical Observer* as 'puerile' and 'feeble and ill executed'. At the same time, he confessed himself chagrined that it had met with apathy from the medical profession, whom he accused of self-interest in the continuance of the patent remedy trade, for the dangerous cases from which they made their own living were often caused by injudicious use of such products. More usefully, however, Clayton gave an insight into Butler's methods of gathering endorsements.

From Col. RIDDELL, *Exmouth, Devonshire,*
To Messrs. CHING & BUTLER, Cheapside, *London*.

GENTLEMEN,—Having seen many honouralbe testimonies of the efficacy of CHING's WORM LOZENGES, I was induced to make trial of them; for, from a twenty-two years residence in the East-Indies, I had for a long time been subject to a liver complaint, and violent bilious obstructions; to remove which, every other medicine had proved ineffectual : but after taking a few doses of your PATENT WORM LOZENGES, I found myself considerably relieved ; and by continuing their use, have received essential benefit ; and whenever I feel any return of the former symptoms, I have recourse to it, which invariably removes my complaints. I have since given your medicine to my own children, and to many of my acquaintance ; also to numbers of the poor in my neighbourhood, and in no one instance have I known it fail of success ; and in several cases, I might say, it has performed miraculous cures ; and indeed I have received such abundant and remarkable proofs of its singular efficacy, that too much cannot be said in its praise. I shall feel a personal pleasure in recommending your CHING's WORM LOZENGES for the removal of bilious obstructions, or any complaint on the liver.

And remain, Gentlemen, yours. &c.
Exmouth. February 10, 1802.   JOHN RIDDELL.

Sold wholesale and retail, at Mr. Butler's, No. 4. Cheapside, corner of Paternoster-row ; and retail by Peck, printer. and E. Browne, Hull ; Wolstenholme, York ; Sheardown, Doncaster; Binns, Leeds ; Drury, and Drummond, Lincoln ; and most medicine venders, booksellers, and perfumers, in every town ; in boxes at 2s. 9d. To prevent counterfeits, his Majesty's Honourable Commissioners have been pleased to order the name of R. Butler, to be engraved in black on the stamp, which stamp is affixed around each box.

Where may also be had,
Gamble's British Herb Tea, Tobacco, and Snuff.
Ching and Butler's Ginger Seeds.
Ford's Balsam of Horehound, for Coughs, &c.
Dixon's Antibilious Pills, &c. &c.

Ching's Worm Lozenges. *Hull Packet, Tuesday 7 August 1804. Image*
Image reproduced with kind permission of the British Newspaper Archive
(www.britishnewspaperarchive.co.uk)

In 1800, Messrs Smart and Cowslade, Chemists, of Reading, forwarded to Ching and Butler a testimonial they had received from a local father, Richard Bitmead, who had been to their shop and 'related the particulars with tears of gratitude in his eyes'. Bitmead's son had suffered swollen legs and red spots all over his body, attended with pains and sickness that reduced him to a 'perfect skeleton'. As the child sank towards the very maw of death, someone recommended Ching's Worm Lozenges, and 'on giving him the first dose, he was immediately freed from pains, and voided a great quantity of filth, resembling worms in a putrid state'.

Further doses brought forth 'a quantity of slimy green matter', after which the perfect skeleton became the epitome of perfect health. Yet such a miracle proved spurious. M.J. Clayton claimed to have a letter from the chemist, Mr Cowslade, admitting that he had been requested to write the testimonial himself at Butler's instruction.

Other endorsements, the *Medical Observer* discovered, were genuine but used without the permission of their writers. The Lord Chief Baron of the Exchequer, Sir Archibald Macdonald, reported that his child was 'delivered of a load which cannot with propriety be described, but which appeared to be the NEST of these pernicious animals'. Macdonald recommended the lozenges to his buddy, the Bishop of Carlisle, whose son derived similar benefit. The Baron and the Bishop both wrote glowing reports of the treatment, but were not amused to find their testimonials appearing for years to come in Butler's advertisements.

The worthy personages were perhaps naïve in communicating their satisfaction with the product, but their involvement shows the indistinctness of the line between orthodox and proprietary medicine. Macdonald and Carlisle had both used the Worm Lozenges under the supervision of their family doctors, who were aware of the ingredients and able to monitor the dosage. They did not see the lozenges as a 'quack remedy' but as one of many forms in which it was acceptable to administer mercury as a vermifuge. They were also under the impression that John Ching (still alive at the time) was a qualified apothecary and they could not have predicted the product's growth as a patent medicine under Butler's misleading claims about its safety.

M.J. Clayton, in his enthusiasm to 'dispel the noxious vapours of empiricism, and hurl the hydra-headed monster "down to its native hell"', was appalled at how the lozenges' reputation had become 'intrenched behind the sacred name of a Christian Minister! Or the prostituted recommendation of a British Peer!' His campaigning, however, had limited reach and Ching's Worm Lozenges remained on sale for the best part of another century.

Clayton's own two children had narrowly escaped the same fate as his nephew Thomas, one of them ending up so damaged by the lozenges that he would 'carry the marks of their ravages to the grave'. Whatever the literary merit of the *Essay*, it is infused with parental feeling and a rage against the fraudulent claims that could leave anyone – not just the gullible or stupid – bereft. Its chilling curse on Butler clearly came from the heart:

> Dire conscience all thy guilty dreams affright,
> With the most solemn horrors of the night.
> The screams of infants ever fill thy ears,
> And injured heav'n be deaf to all thy prayers.

15

MAKING THE PATIENT A PERFECT FRIGHT

I called at the dentist today, according to my appointment. He
recommends passing a thread of silk between my teeth every day and
brushing my decayed teeth with spirits.

A polished brass plate and a fashionably decorated treatment
room awaited the well-to-do dental patient of the 1830s,
but at the time the young diarist Anthony Evans braved the
perennial advice to floss, there were no guarantees about the
quality of treatment.

Dentistry was unregulated and any enterprising fellow
could set up shop without having pulled a tooth in his life.
For the more skilled practitioner, who would normally
have qualified as a surgeon before specialising in teeth, these
untrained people were unwelcome rivals. Not only did they
give dentistry a bad name (which some surgeons were quite
capable of doing for themselves) but they possessed the self-
promotional effrontery to earn a lot more money.

Surgeon-dentist C. Bene, writing to *The Lancet* in 1833,
related the story of a baronet plagued with toothache. 'Sir
D.H.B.' stopped his curricle at a smart house on London's
New Road where 'Teeth Extracted' gleamed in gold lettering
in the window. He entered, seeking relief from his pain.

The 'dentist', after some fidgeting and shuffling about the room, took a survey of the decayed tooth, but it was not until he had been frequently spurred on by the importunities of his patient with 'Come, come, for God's sake, make haste and ease me,' that he commenced the apparently important operation.

The extraction complete, the dentist 'began to jump about the shop like one overjoyed at some fortunate event'. He admitted that he had started his business that very day and the baronet's tooth was the first he had ever drawn.

Two years later, another *Lancet* correspondent described a case that left less cause for celebration. An 8-year-old girl's permanent lower incisors came through before her milk teeth had fallen out. An itinerant practitioner describing himself as dentist to the King of Holland asserted that she had a double row of teeth (a circumstance he had often encountered before) and extracted the permanent ones. When the tooth fairy finally visited, the unfortunate little girl was left with an expanse of gum.

Conscientious dentists despaired at the extent of quackery, but those who expressed their opinions in the medical journals were isolated voices in a fragmented profession. Although dentistry had emerged as a sole occupation, 'surgeon-dentists' (a title that could be adopted by anyone) were still relatively few in number. Tooth extraction also formed part of a general surgeon's role, an extra service offered by chemists, or a sideline to unrelated occupations. New inventions and methods did not take hold on a wide scale – individuals kept them secret as a way of enhancing their own reputation and income. In addition, surgical proficiency did not make someone capable of crafting artificial teeth, while mechanical dentists from an artisan background might create good dentures but have no surgical training. Little solidarity existed between, or even within, these groups.

In 1852, for example, a dispute broke out between two inexperienced practitioners over a terrible set of false teeth, illustrating just how easy it was to set up in practice. A Trowbridge chemist, Mr Parker, began to advertise that after much painstaking study he had become a surgeon–dentist, able to supply artificial teeth that would restore the wearer's beauty and be indistinguishable from the real thing. His problems began when a customer placed an order and it became apparent that he would actually have to learn how to make teeth, or at least find someone who could. He called in a mechanical dentist named Mr Ballinger from Bath, agreeing to pay him £7 15s for a set of dentures, for which he would charge the patient £12.

Ballinger and Parker visited the customer to take an impression of her mouth, but they needn't have bothered as the resulting set of teeth bore no relation to it: 'The lady's mouth would not close; the front teeth were all inside of the jaw, and eating or speaking was out of the question.'

They returned the next day with an amended attempt, but this proved even less successful: 'In addition to the mouth being kept wider open than before, the teeth stuck out like so many tusks, making the patient a perfect fright.'

Having had the teeth shoved into her mouth in a manner that was 'truly pitiable', the lady refused to buy them from Parker; Parker refused to pay Ballinger for them so Ballinger took the chemist to court.

Another mechanical dentist, who appeared as witness, had also been approached by Parker to make teeth for his customers. This elderly man, John Wood, at least had some experience – he had made no fewer than eighteen sets for himself and wore a different one each day. He proved this to the court by whipping out his false teeth and holding them up, saying, 'Now look, look at me!' Observers were astonished to see that 'the old man's nose and chin almost met when deprived of his teeth'.

Wood's evidence does not seem to have added much to the proceedings beyond entertainment, but a more reputable dentist examined the dentures made by Ballinger and discovered that all the teeth, whether front or back, were the same. They 'displayed on the part of the maker total ignorance of the practice of dentistry'.

Ballinger admitted that he was not a dentist, but a jeweller who had lately started making false teeth. Neither he nor the defendant emerged from the episode well, and the magistrate declined to send the case before a jury, ordering both participants to pay their own costs.

More principled practitioners were well aware of such problems and during the 1840s, individuals such as George Waite and James Robinson called for organisation and official qualifications. Although these attempts met with little success, the issues became open for public discussion. The first British dental journal appeared in 1843 – it did not last long, but its successor, *Forceps*, campaigned for regulation, lamenting that:

> In this country any quack who chooses to place a brass plate on his door, some artificial masticators in his window, and advertises his list of charges in the papers is a dentist to all intents and purposes.

Mr Bene's anecdote about the baronet might have been embellished to support his views, but it illustrates a factor in the success of unqualified dentists – the urgency of agony. Toothache is equally excruciating for baronet or pauper and the desperate individual could not spare days comparing the certificates and experience of various practitioners. If you can't eat because a pulsating tooth abscess is driving you up the wall, the long-term ideal of a unified dental profession is not your first priority.

Although pain is a great leveller, social status did make a difference to dental health. John Gray, a surgeon who published a tract on *Dental Advice* in 1836 and an expanded version,

Dental Practice, in 1837, observed that the teeth of the upper classes were worse than those of labourers. He attributed this to their habit of visiting fashionable dentists – who became fashionable through chutzpah rather than ability.

> In the higher ranks of society it is scarcely possible to find a person of the age of twenty-four who has not lost some teeth, and so many of the remainder are so stopped with gold, that their mouths have some resemblance to the window of a jeweller's shop.

Comparing the local trade directory with the list of members of the Royal College of Surgeons, Gray found that only 7 out of more than 120 surgeon-dentists had surgical qualifications. His views on quackery did not, however, prevent him using his pamphlet to advertise his own proprietary dentifrice and tincture, which boasted an endorsement from Sir Humphrey Davy.

Gray believed that the state of the nation's gnashers was worse than it had been in the eighteenth century when they were largely left alone. He accused quack dentists of ruining people's teeth by clasping false ones to the real ones and by treating young people's overcrowded teeth by filing between them – a process that destroyed the enamel and caused food to get trapped in the gaps, leading to sensitivity and decay.

While the poor did not necessarily go around with full pearly-white smiles, the lack of such interference at least gave their teeth a chance of remaining sound for longer. But when emergencies arose, dental services were accessible even to those with little money. Some dentists allocated part of their working day to the treatment of the poor and in 1839 the charitable London Institution for Diseases of the Teeth was established.

The diarist Anthony Evans's appointment with his floss-loving dentist came at a time when a practitioner could be proficient and well-educated, a charlatan trying out a new money-making scheme, or anything in between. Change, however, was brewing. Reputable practitioners would agitate for the formalisation of their profession and dentistry took to the chair to undergo an agonisingly long-drawn-out process of reform.

16

LYING ROUND WITH BASINS BY THEIR HEADS

Mer-Syren: a name imbued with the mystery of the deep, evoking a glimpse of a shimmering tail-fin gliding beneath the waves. Could this be a magical remedy infused with the glitter of a syren's golden hair? Was it concocted from a rare species of seaweed whose powers could cure every disease? Or was Mer-Syren as fake as Barnum's famed Feejee Mermaid, half-monkey, half-fish, whose desiccated body had once enthralled the public?

The name might have held all the romance of the open ocean, but the reality of Mer-Syren was firmly rooted in the land.

The product began life as a cure for seasickness. With transatlantic travel booming at the turn of the twentieth century, the issue of *mal de mer* was pertinent yet difficult to address. Seasoned travellers advocated methods that had worked for them, but no effective medical cure was available. If a proprietary remedy such as Mer-Syren could be found to work, its inventor could expect to travel first class for the rest of his life. As Singapore paper the *Straits Times* put it:

> Who was ever properly seasick who would not promptly sacrifice all his worldly goods – sweetheart, parents, kindred friends – for a sure and prompt recovery? With a single gallon of such a remedy, a stonehearted blackmailer on some such ocean palace as the *Lucania*

could make a fortune out of the afflicted millionaires during one trip across the Atlantic.

Seasickness, then as now, was miserable and undignified. In 1870, American physician Benjamin Fordyce Barker described a typical crossing of the English Channel that would not be unfamiliar to the modern passenger: 'I should advise one not to go down into the cabin below, where the sight of those lying round, with basins by their heads, is of itself exceedingly provocative to the sensitive stomach.'

With limited options for rehydration, however, and with existing medical conditions under unreliable control, seasickness was not just unpleasant but potentially fatal. And it was not only the long ocean voyages that posed a risk. In 1902, Eliza Farries, who had a heart condition and diabetes, took a boat trip round the coast from Eastbourne to Brighton – a distance of some 26 miles – and was severely sick, dying on the return journey. The same route also waved off Mrs Williamson Carter Gray, who died of heart failure in 1909 following the exhaustion of continued vomiting.

Physicians' advice focused on prevention. Fordyce Barker advised eating a hearty meal before the voyage (presumably something delicious so as to make its resurgence more palatable), board the ship early and get everything you need within reach, then go to bed before it sets off. One should eat regularly, but without raising the head for the first couple of days, and once acclimatised to the motion of the ship, only get up after having some porridge or sea-biscuit. This was no doubt more practical for cabin passengers than those in steerage.

Other methods of prevention sought to minimise the disharmony between visual signals and those experienced by the other senses. Dr G. Arbour Stephens of Glasgow advocated keeping one eye closed or covered – perhaps pirates had the right idea all along. The Italian ambassador in Washington,

Edmondo Mayor des Planches, was said to have cured his own seasickness by spending the voyage looking at his reflection in a mirror. He discovered this method by accident, having struggled up from his berth just to check how bad he looked, and finding that he instantly felt well enough to tuck in to a substantial breakfast. A different method originating in Italy was a curative belt consisting of a triangular pad that pressed against the hollow of the stomach. Designed by Dr Calliano of Turin, it featured 'an amusing little screw' to increase the pressure.

By 1909, ship's surgeon John W. Dougall of the *Carthaginian* was reporting success with hypnosis, but there was still plenty of room on the market for a quick-acting, convenient remedy that could easily be purchased before embarking.

Into the search for this elusive cure came Mer-Syren, beginning life in Singapore around 1905. It had the impressive credential of being created by a respected and experienced seafarer – Captain Arthur Neagle, a Londoner in command of the Eastern Extension, Australasia and China Telegraph Company's steamer, the *Recorder*. The ship had the heroic job of repairing damaged undersea cables, often battling tough weather conditions to reopen communication between nations. In 1907, 34-year-old Captain Neagle got married and settled down at Westcliff-on-Sea in Essex to devote his attention to the sale of his invention. Attractive pictorial advertisements promised an 'instantaneous remedy'. A testimonial from indigestion sufferer J.P. Thompson reported that 'a few minutes after taking the first powder I felt relieved, and in an hour I was perfectly well'. His symptoms had 'vanish[ed] like magic'.

Such claims attracted the attention of the British Medical Association, which included Mer-Syren in its series of investigations into advertised remedies. First published in the *British Medical Journal* in June 1911, the report appeared in the

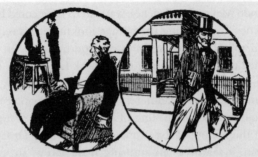

A late night at your club is frequently followed by an attack of <u>Biliousness</u>.

There is only <u>one cure</u> for this most distressing complaint and that is

MER-SYREN
Powders

Neither drug nor purgative—<u>tasteless</u>, <u>soothing.</u> They make you fit by morning.

"One dose, one cure" explains in a nutshell the efficacy of "Mer-Syren" Powders, which have <u>Never been known to Fail.</u>

From all Chemists and Druggists, in boxes, 2/9, or direct, post free, from The MER-SYREN CO., 17. Cockspur St., London, S.W.

Mer-Syren Powders. *Manchester Courier and Lancashire General Advertiser, Friday 12 November 1909. Image © Northcliffe Media Limited. Image created courtesy of THE BRITISH LIBRARY BOARD. Image reproduced with kind permission of the British Newspaper Archive (www.britishnewspaperarchive.co.uk)*

book *More Secret Remedies: What they cost and what they contain* the following year, and it was here that Mer-Syren's contents came to public knowledge.

The *BMJ* gave extensive quotations from a promotional booklet, 'How the body cures itself' by someone named Dr Pearson, who had supposedly been Principal Medical Officer at North Bhangalpore in India. It read:

> Mer-Syren is composed of the active principles of certain rare plants which flourish in the valleys situated on the southern slopes of the Himalayas, between the immense gorge separating Nepal from Bhutan on the East, and the Almorah on the North West.

While the exotic location imbued the product with an aura of Eastern mystery, it was also suitably inaccessible for the average British consumer. Sceptics would have to have a lot of time and money to prove these rare plants were non-existent. Even their names, the booklet said, were unknown to Western science, and could not, therefore, be found in any pharmacopoeia. Pre-empting the possibility of anyone investigating the ingredients, the author stated that 'the alkaloids on which its extraordinary and startling effects depend cannot be determined by analysis, as all organic substances defy detection by any means known to chemical science'.

That did not stop the BMA analysing it and discovering that its contents were more likely to be found in Westcliff-on-Sea than the hidden valleys of the Himalayas.

Oddly, because the *BMJ* writer could not find Bhangalpore in the maps section of the *Encyclopaedia Britannica*, he implied that it was not a real place. To be fair to the proprietor of Mer-Syren, however, Bhangalpore was an old name for Bhagalpur in Bengal, a significant centre of trade since the days of the East India Company. In 1901 the district had a population of more than 2,088,000 and its main administrative centre, the town of Bhagalpur, was providing revenue for the British crown through a variety of industries including silk and cloth production. Whether a Dr Pearson had been Principal Medical Officer there was perhaps more doubtful. His opinion of his own profession was uncomplimentary and he held the view that the modern Materia Medica was based on 'beetles, spider's webs, crab's eyes, tiger's tongue, rhinoceros' horn, and other repulsive objects'. Medicine, he informed the public, had barely progressed since the days of William Harvey, the sixteenth-century physician who first described the circulation of the blood. Diseases were 'arranged in a few haphazard groups, as motley and incongruous in their composition and disposition as the various sections of, say, a political party'.

Mer-Syren's focus on seasickness was shortlived and its scope soon expanded to appeal to even the most determined landlubber. Digestive complaints, liver conditions and the various vague symptoms associated with them would immediately succumb to its powers.

For indigestion and dyspepsia, the dose was two powders placed dry on the tongue and washed down with hot water. For bilious headaches, which included instances of 'the morning after the night before', one powder was sufficient (unless you had really been going for it) and should be taken with cold water. Mer-Syren later became available in tablet form too.

In 1911 the Mer-Syren Company went into voluntary liquidation and was regurgitated as Mer-Syren (1911) Ltd. Its claims became more exaggerated – ailments such as nervous dyspepsia and 'brain dulness' owed their existence to a poisonous gas present in the system. Mer-Syren 'absolutely gets rid of this blood, nerve and brain poisoning gas in 10 minutes, afterwards cleaning out of the system the delayed waste-matters that are the cause of the trouble'.

Although Mer-Syren would permeate every part of the body, enabling the consumer to feel its good effects all over, it also held the power to target whichever organ was 'in any way deranged, or whose structures may be breaking down in consequence of disease'. This remained a completely natural process far removed from the harsh drugs beloved of the medical profession. Each dose of Mer-Syren was a '10-Minute Health Lesson', teaching the consumer the right way to look after his or her body. Potential customers could send off for a trial dose which, according to the testimonials, was enough to have a dramatic effect. 'I AM DELIGHTED TO SAY I AM A DIFFERENT MAN,' boomed F. White of Nottingham after using his free sample.

Some of Mer-Syren's claims, however, were true. A primary selling point was that the product was 'not an opiate, purgative or drug, and is perfectly harmless, being of vegetable origin'. This proved to be correct when the BMA's analysis found Mer-Syren to contain powdered potato and nothing more.

Had the well-travelled Captain Neagle genuinely discovered a plant in the East only to turn to a more accessible ingredient back home? Or, having had plentiful opportunity to observe the psychological component of seasickness, did he recognise the value of a placebo? Wisely, he had not trumpeted his name and background in the promotion of Mer-Syren, and went on to continue his career as a sea captain, and later a shipbroker, without his patent medicine associations causing any apparent detriment to his good reputation.

Whatever his intentions, it was fitting that the sufferers from the awful *mal de mer* should gain hope from the humble *pomme de terre*.

17

A PLACE WHERE URINE
WAS KEPT

The trouble with creating a web of deception is that you need a good memory. Not only did the Bennett brothers have to recall their patients' names and faces, but they also had to keep track of their own. Their promises to cure deafness made them more than £4,000 a year, but it was a precarious business and one that they must be ready to abandon at a moment's notice.

A deaf person seeking treatment in 1850s London had plenty of options. He or she could consult Surgeon Coulston, Dr Watters, Dr Matton, Dr Singleton, Dr Skinner, Dr Brandon, or attend the British and Foreign Ear Infirmary at 32 Spring Gardens. But in the event of being dissatisfied with your treatment and consulting more than one of these practitioners, chances are you would find them strangely familiar. And if you knew what was in their medicine, you would not want it anywhere near your ears.

Multiple ads under different names were a mid-nineteenth-century scam also common among the spermatorrhoea gangs mentioned in Chapter 5. No patient was obliged to remain loyal to a single practitioner, qualified or otherwise, so when one treatment didn't work, it was well within their power to try another … and another, until all funds or options were exhausted. The trick for the medical fraudster was to be behind as many of these options as possible, taking the same victim's money time and again.

The gang operated under the leadership of John Gibson Bennett, who in 1859 was around 40 years old. His younger brother William was in partnership with him and there was also some involvement for a third brother, Henry. These former card-sharpers were backed up by a team of questionable characters, including a qualified surgeon named John Watters, their ultimately disloyal 'chief assistant', Claude Edwards, and a tame attorney, Ambrose Haynes.

The Bennetts adopted several tactics to ensure patients did not see the same brother under more than one name. Their premises at Spring Gardens sported a series of mirrors giving a good view of anyone approaching the door. A servant would welcome the patient in, asking whether he or she had previously consulted other practitioners – naming a few to jog their memory if necessary. Once alone amid the gold-and-crimson décor of the consulting room, the patient might feel as though they were being watched. A hole in the door allowed the Bennetts to see who was in there and decide which of them should pose as the doctor.

Things could become complicated. In December 1857, a patient recognised the servant who admitted her. The servant managed to pretend he had formerly been assistant to another doctor and was now working for 'Dr Watters', but it was clear to him that the patient was going to be familiar with John G. Bennett. What were they to do, since the other Bennett brothers were not around? Fortunately, the lawyer Ambrose Haynes happened to be visiting.

'Will you oblige me, my dear fellow?' Bennett allegedly said to the lawyer, 'Go and see this woman, as Dr Watters, it won't take you a moment.' According to the servant, Haynes did oblige, taking two guineas from the woman for some medicine. Haynes, however, who insisted that he was not connected with the Bennetts in any other capacity than as their lawyer, avoided prosecution.

The treatment itself was similarly complex. Claude Edwards, the assistant involved in making the medicines, identified five components of the system – ear-drops, embrocation, injection, fumigation and tincture. The basic ingredient of each, however, was the same – urine. Sometimes patients also received a box of powder, namely sawdust.

Under the Bennetts' treatment, ears were bombarded with urine from every direction. The injection fluid for syringing the ears comprised sugar of lead, zinc sulphate and urine. The embrocation, which the patient was to rub on the nape of the neck and behind the ears before bed, contained oil, ammonia and urine. The fumigation, which involved a vapour bath in the form of a tin box with a tube at the top, costing £2 10s, offered the added danger of burns. A patient, Joseph Woolrich, described how he had been instructed to use it:

> I had six bottles to put into this, and had some wool to put in; and I was to buy some tincture of myrrh, and while it was burning, I was to put the tube into my ear for seven or eight minutes each time, twisting a paper up in my ear to prevent the tube being too hot for the skin.

All these details came out because the Bennetts didn't manage to keep one step ahead of patient power. In 1857, a young woman called Mary Scattergood visited 'Surgeon Coulston' in response to an advert that promised a cure in ten minutes. She soon discovered that this came at the extortionate price of 10 guineas, which she could not afford, but she agreed to pay 5 on the proviso that a hearing apparatus was part of the deal. She expected to undergo some procedure that would have an immediate effect, but 'Coulston' sent her away with a bottle of mixture instead. By the next morning, he told her, she would certainly be cured – though he continued with less certainty by saying, 'Use it again the following night in case you are not.'

The mixture gave Miss Scattergood sore ears and a headache – added to which, she had never got the apparatus she paid for, so she returned to Coulston's premises. He wasn't there, and his assistant (who considerably resembled him) said he had gone away for a few days.

Miss Scattergood called again several times but the assistant at last told her Coulston had gone to Madeira, so she had to wave goodbye to her 5 guineas and put this one down to experience. It wasn't until two years later, when she accompanied a friend to an ear-doctor called Dr Matton (or Dr Watters according to some reports), that she discovered it was the same fellow – and this time she wasn't going to let him get away with it.

William Bennett recognised Miss Scattergood and made a rapid exit, but she had seen enough. She had the older Bennett summoned to Westminster County Court, and other witnesses came forward to testify that he had conned them too – one man told how Bennett had called him a 'grey-headed old rascal' and threatened to throw him down the stairs.

John G. Bennett, who 'wore a moustache, and appeared to be about 40 years old', denied everything, claiming never to have seen Miss Scattergood in his life. William, who also wore a moustache and was about ten years younger, tried to pin the blame on the non-existent Surgeon Coulston, but the judge ruled in favour of Miss Scattergood – she got back her 5 guineas and John G. Bennett was indicted for perjury.

He didn't turn up to his hearing at Bow Street Police Court, but some interesting evidence came out. The London Medical Registration Association, which had helped Miss Scattergood bring Bennett to trial, analysed Bennett's mixture and found it to comprise urine and alum. A former porter to the gang told of a 'place where urine was kept' and that he had helped to make up the bottles.

Claude Edwards was by this time claiming to regret ever having worked for the Bennetts. He recalled an incident where William Bennett had left him to rub embrocation onto a patient's back while Bennett went to the pub for a couple of glasses of brandy and water. On his return, he confided in Edwards: 'I think I must let Mr King off for twelve guineas, but if I can drop it into him for more I will.' Mr King ended up paying more than £30 for what he thought was a traditional remedy discovered by 'Dr Watters' in China or Japan.

The magistrate issued a warrant for the arrest of the two older Bennett brothers, but by then their whereabouts 'appeared somewhat uncertain'.

When Ambrose Haynes was tried and acquitted for the fraud of impersonating Dr Watters, Edwards continued to present himself as a beleaguered employee just getting on with his job. Speaking of compounding the medicines, he said:

> the whole of us assisted – as servants we were bound to do it – I did not think it was honest, I thought it was great roguery – I advised John Gibson Bennett against it many times – I went on with it for two years, because John Gibson Bennett repeatedly said he would establish Dr. Watters in legitimate practice, and we were to have a share – I continued acting like a rogue for two years, in hopes of going honestly at last.

When not in front of a judge, however, Edwards's hope of going straight proved less ardent. Taking the Bennetts' hasty departure as a money-making opportunity, he stripped 32 Spring Gardens of its contents, right down to the mirrors warning of patients' approach. He was disgruntled when Thomas Oldfield, the Bennetts' former porter, ran off with a gun that he had asked him to look after. Edwards, however, reconsidered his attempts to prosecute Oldfield for theft on the basis that the gun actually belonged to neither of them.

The Bennetts had vacated a niche in the market for deafness cures and Claude Edwards was just the person to fill it. He and John Nichol Watters, who until then had only been on the periphery of the business, established a new ear infirmary at 28 Mount Gardens and used the same methods as before to treat patients.

Watters held qualifications from 'College and Hall', meaning he had a diploma from the Royal College of Surgeons of London and was also a licensed apothecary. People with these certificates were termed 'general practitioners' and although they were not university-trained doctors, they were the providers of orthodox medical care most likely to be consulted by the average person, particularly outside the cities.

Certificates, however, were no guarantee of moral fibre. Back in 1831, when he was in his early twenties, this sporter of 'a little moustache and rather carroty whiskers' had spent time in gaol for inciting someone to arson.

He and a trusted friend, medical student Richard Steele, wanted to go to France to study anatomy, but lacked the funds to do so. Watters suggested an insurance job on his premises, for which his friend would receive £108. Steele could use the proceeds to set up his own shop and insure it to the hilt; Watters would then return the favour and burn it down. There was no time to lose. In dialogue worthy of a stage villain, Watters told Steele: 'A secret long hatched gets wind – we must do it to-night.'

Steele agreed to the plot but went straight to the police, who accompanied him to Watters' shop at the appointed time and found combustible materials arranged as Watters had promised. The surgeon was imprisoned for eighteen months, and presumably no longer considered Steele a trusted friend.

In 1859, however, all this was behind him. He and Claude Edwards syringed, embrocated and fumigated ears until the day a patient expressed surprise at his bill and went to borrow the money from a friend, returning with Police Inspector Young. The aurists each went to prison for eighteen months.

The Bennett brothers, however, continued to lie low and avoid prosecution. Their names and faces disappeared to places unknown, and with them, the stale smell of their fraudulent remedies.

18

TO AVOID ALL APPEARANCE
OF PUFFING

Though overshadowed by the flamboyant mountebank, eclipsed by the moustachioed conman and bereft of an advertising budget, the more humble maker of remedies could still carve out a niche in the market.

Phoebe Blaste of Eign Street, Hereford, was part of what modern politicians might call a 'hard-working family'. She would not have dreamt of taking to the stage and delivering a harangue about the miraculousness of her cures and she did not claim to possess a sheaf of medical degrees from foreign universities. Instead, she produced her medicine at home and sold it by the quart to a local and loyal customer base. Word of mouth formed the main vehicle for its promotion, but on occasions during the 1830s and 1840s she placed advertisements in the local papers – advertisements that now give a glimpse into a side of the proprietary medicine trade that blurred the line between home remedy and commercial product.

Mrs Blaste's medicine started life as Clarke's Herbaceous Liquid, compounded 'chiefly from British herbs' and the product of a recipe handed down by her father, Thomas Clarke of Frodsham in Cheshire. Phoebe moved to Hereford when she married Nathaniel Blaste in 1815, and her husband became the official proprietor of the Liquid, advertising it by means of testimonials:

> Thomas Williams, of the Above Eign, in the parish of All Saints, in the
> City of Hereford, declares, that being out and having caught a violent
> cold, which had materially affected his breath and lungs, he was
> recommended to take Clarke's Herbaceous Liquid; and after taking
> two bottles was effectually restored and continues in good health.

With a day job as a groom, Nathaniel had a ready-made
market for selling the Herbaceous Liquid as a cure for animal
diseases, and when Phoebe became the named proprietor of
the remedy in around 1833, she advertised it 'for the CURE
OF DISORDERS incident to CATTLE, HORSES, SHEEP
etc.' Luckily for the Liquid's reputation, some of these disorders
could resolve naturally. For 'murrain', a tick-borne parasitic
disease causing dark-coloured urine in cattle, the dose was a
quarter of a pint of Liquid in a pint of warm ale twice a day.
Mild cases would appear to be responding to this treatment
even though it is likely they would have improved anyway.

The dose for a 'loin-fallen' cow, meanwhile, was three
tablespoonsful in a pint of warm ale twice a day, 'the beast
afterwards being rubbed across the loins for half an hour with
the Liquid'.

'Loin-fallen' was a colloquial term for milk fever, a condition
with dramatic symptoms of paralysis now known to result from
low calcium levels in a cow that has recently calved and begun
producing milk. In the period when Clarke's Herbaceous
Liquid was available, the involvement of hypocalcaemia in milk
fever was unknown and the prognosis was poor, but some cases
did recover perfectly. In 1853, for example, W.A. Cartwright
MRCVS, one of the earliest professional veterinary surgeons,
attended a cow showing typical symptoms – she had difficulty
walking and ended up flat out on the ground, moaning and
suffering a distended abdomen.

Cartwright's methods of treatment, in line with the common
practice of the time, were aggressive. As well as administering a

purging medicine and rubbing brandy and mustard on the cow's loins, Cartwright applied blisters to her back and later 'poured some hot water along the spine from a tea kettle, and she was evidently sensible to the application, as it gave her great pain and made her turn over on the other side'. After two days of being unable to get up, the cow stood and 'was soon all right again'. Readers familiar with the representation of the veterinary profession in popular culture need not be disappointed; Cartwright also performed the inevitable. 'On passing my hand up the rectum, I withdrew a quantity of hardened faeces.'

Other cases involved bloodletting, turpentine enemas and draughts of ammonia and brandy, but recovery was largely dependent on how severe the case had been in the first place. A seemingly half-dead cow managing to get up and suckle her calf was an affecting testimony to whatever treatment had most recently been given. If a remedy like Clarke's Herbaceous Liquid happened to coincide with this heartwarming scene, word could spread quickly and the product's reputation be secured.

Half an hour is an awfully long time to spend rubbing a cow's loins. A small bottle of the Liquid wouldn't be up to the job, so Mrs Blaste sold it by the quart for 7s. But the Herbaceous Liquid was a versatile product, suited for the ills of humans as well as those of beasts. It was:

> justly celebrated for curing all complaints in the Breast and Stomach, Rheumatism, Scurvy, Pains of the Back, Loins, Typhus Fever, Chincough &c. By applying it immediately to a burn or a scald, it prevents blister. It is also most excellent for the Gravel, and a certain cure for the Rheumatic gout, even when the Joints and Sinews are contracted.

In spite of the panacean qualities of their product, the Blastes did not have world domination in mind. They advertised infrequently and close to home, sticking to the newspapers of

Hereford and otherwise relying on customers to spread the word. Even their testimonials were from a narrow area – those included in one advert in 1824, for example, were both from the parish of All Saints, where the Blastes themselves lived. But far from being a case of getting their chums to endorse the Liquid, this localised support suggests respect for the product's qualities and some genuine belief that it worked. If the Blastes had been out to con people with a useless or dangerous medicine, they would soon have come to grief. Any dissatisfied customers knew exactly where they lived.

Nathaniel Blaste died in December 1842, his standing in the community reflected by a touching announcement in the *Hereford Times*: 'Deeply regretted, aged 60 years, Mr Nathaniel Blast, of this city. He was a worthy, honest and industrious man, and very much respected.'

Phoebe Blaste's own health was not good and for a few years the Herbaceous Liquid had to take a lower priority in her life. When she relaunched it in 1845, the product had a new, catchier name – 'The Life's Friend' – and its focus was on human illnesses, including insanity and consumption.

According to the adverts, Mrs Blaste herself had suffered three strokes, or 'fits of apoplexy', and recovered thanks to her own medicine. In spite of the new name and elevated claims, however, Mrs Blaste still appears reticent about blowing her own trumpet, deciding not to include any testimonials out of 'the wish to avoid all appearance of puffing'. She was almost apologetic about not having had the chance to make any medicine: 'Inability to devote the time and attention necessary to its preparation, has alone prevented the proprietress from bringing it before the public in a more prominent manner.'

Phoebe Blaste died in London in 1853 and her two daughters do not appear to have continued production of The Life's Friend. The remedy's existence is now only known because Mrs Blaste left behind some evidence of having promoted it.

Otherwise, demand for it was down to 'the recommendations of those who have experienced its wonderful curative powers'.

It is impossible to know how many other ordinary people made at least part of their living from small-scale production of medicines at home, but it's clear that the history of commercial remedies isn't just a story of fraud and gullibility. It suited Phoebe Blaste to sell The Life's Friend and it suited her customers to buy it. Can't say fairer than that.

19

ALL CAME ABOUT AS I DESIRED

The name 'Thomasso's Magic Female Pills' has a sense of the theatrical about it. Redolent of the warmth and light of the music hall, it evokes the image of a flamboyant Italian conjuror delighting his audience with feats of prestidigitation. The remedy itself might not have been magical, but it was part of a tradition of secrecy and linguistic sleight of hand.

Advertised in the 1890s, Thomasso's Magic Female Pills claimed to be 'the acknowledged Leading Remedy for correcting all irregularities and removing obstructions of whatever cause'. They had a lot of competition. The decade saw a proliferation of advertisements for similar 'female' remedies, whose proprietors were careful to present them as cures for 'stoppage of the menses'. But in healthy, sexually active young women, unexplained amenorrhoea was too rare to have kept even one patent medicine proprietor in business. In 1898, *The Lancet* made enquiries of the gynaecology department of a London hospital and learnt that of 183 female patients who did not menstruate, 12 had long-term known causes, 12 were pre-pubescent and 156 (96.5 per cent) were pregnant. 'Stoppage of the menses' was a euphemism whose meaning was clear to the intended market for female pills – the 'obstruction' they promised to terminate was a foetus.

These products and their customers trod on dangerous ground. Abortion was a criminal offence and the maximum sentence for attempting it – whether successfully or not – was a lifetime of penal servitude. Yet for an unmarried servant facing the loss of her income, accommodation and reputation, or for an exhausted and impoverished mother already trying to feed too many mouths, the consequences of an unwanted pregnancy were grim enough to justify the risk.

Weekly penny publications such as the *Illustrated Police News* (voted the 'Worst English Newspaper' by readers of the *Pall Mall Gazette* in 1886, but deservedly popular for its sensational stories and lively illustrations) carried advertisements for female pills alongside remedies for lost manhood and 'panel-size pictures of French beauties in various positions'.

The language of the advertisements was consistent – they almost always referred to irregularities and obstructions, and their product's efficacy in the most 'obstinate cases'. Some proprietors, such as 'Dr Heseldine', warned enquirers that the medicines 'must not be resorted to for illegal purposes nor on any account be taken by ladies desirous of becoming mothers', simultaneously covering their own backs and hinting at the likely effects. Testimonials, too, indicated the nature of the complaint to be relieved: 'It gives me great pleasure to say that after taking the first bottle of your wonderful medicine all came about as I desired after eleven weeks of misery and anxiety.'

Another implicit means of advertising their purpose was the mention of ingredients traditionally used as abortifacients. Dr Davis's Female Pills, for example, were advertised in 1894 as composed of 'Steel, Pennyroyal, Bitter Apple, Aloes, Pil Cochia ...' To set them apart from similar products, however, they also contained 'other most powerful drugs known only to Dr Davis'. Leonio Thomasso took the opposite tack and claimed that the Magic Female Pills were *not* made from pennyroyal, steel or bitter apple, 'but from drugs far more efficacious'. Both proprietors, however, used these substances as code-words to make their products' purpose clear to potential customers.

Leonio Thomasso (also known as Leoni Tomasso) possibly had an American medical qualification. When he was sued in 1896 by the Society of Apothecaries for practising without a licence, he was able to produce a certificate in Latin from a U.S. university – not that this held any weight with the court, which fined him £20. He also referred to himself on occasions as Dr Thomasso of Ohio. Whether or not this was true, however, he was not entitled to practise as a doctor or pharmacist in the UK. His female pills were part of a range of patent medicines for which he made exaggerated claims.

Thomasso's Health-Restoring Pills for disorders of the stomach, headache, blotches and pimples, were 'the king of pills', superseded by no other. His Perfect Cure was 'the Greatest of all Vital Restoratives' for 'Loss of Nerve Power, from Over Taxed Brain, Grief, Worry, Excesses, &c.' while Thomasso's Lung Healer was 'the best and most wonderful remedy ever offered to the public for the Cure of Coughs, Colds, Asthma, Bronchial Affections, Hoarseness, Wheezing and all Chest Complaints'.

Behind the claims, however, was desperation to sell. Thomasso was heavily in debt and in 1897 he was sued by a newspaper owner for £33-worth of advertising for which he hadn't paid. The newsman pointed out that Thomasso's premises were on the route of the Diamond Jubilee procession and he would therefore coin it by offering seats, and Thomasso was ordered to pay back his debt by £3 a month.

In 1898, *The Lancet* launched an investigation into the reality behind the innocent-sounding language of female pills ads, culminating in an exposé in December that year. Posing as a worried woman of humble station – usually a young unmarried servant but sometimes a 30-year-old wife – *The Lancet* investigators sent off for the various remedies advertised 'To Married Ladies'. On the first contact, they sent the required sum of money and asked for the remedy to be packaged discreetly; if engaging in further correspondence, the fake customer would state outright that she believed herself to be with child.

The orders brought a variety of parcels to *The Lancet*'s assumed addresses, and not always with the discretion requested. A package of Dodd's Female Pills had burst in transit and been decanted into a General Post Office envelope, which could have proved awkward for a genuine customer.

The pills and mixtures underwent analysis, with tests made for dangerous ingredients such as arsenic and mercury. It is possible that the investigators were disappointed to discover that none of the samples contained such poisons, but they published the analyses together with descriptions of the correspondence received from the proprietors.

The remedies were a motley bunch, containing everything from the potentially harmful savin oil to 'a feeble solution of nutmegs and iron'. Dr Davis's Pills, which had claimed to contain numerous well-known abortifacients, were mainly rhubarb and iron scented with oil of roses. Ottey's Pills, meanwhile, were available in three strengths – The Strong, Extra Strong and The Strongest. A printed slip accompanying the standard version suggested: 'If these don't do all you wish, send for the Extra Strong Pills at 5s. 3d., or The Strongest at 10s. per box, and say how far over. If these don't do it the Strongest will shift anything!'

The instructions for Ottey's medicine recommended that 'after success, the pills should be taken regularly', while those for Dr Davis's remedy advised that it be taken 'four or five days before every month' (i.e. before menstruation). The notion of a convenient, ongoing medical form of female contraception was a selling point decades before the introduction of the Pill.

Contraceptive advice and commercial products had been increasingly available since the 1877 trial of Annie Besant and Charles Bradlaugh for republishing an old pamphlet on

For those who live high,
And those who live low,
Thomasso's Pills are a blessing you know.

THOMASSO'S
"Perfect" Pills
ARE THE BEST ON EARTH FOR
Biliousness, Liver complaints, and all Stomach Disorders.

16, Sansom Street, Camberwell. Feb. 27/93.
Mr. Thomasso. Dear Sir.—It gives me much pleasure to add a word of praise to the genuine and sterling qualities of your "Perfect" Pills. They are rightly named, as they are near perfection as possible. . . After trying nearly every pill advertised, I may say there is none to supersede yours for wind, constipation, disordered liver, weak stomach, etc. Compared with others, your pills are par excellence.

I remain, gratefully yours, J. W. Sharp.

Can be ordered through any Chemist at 1/1½, or post free from address below.

The Best Remedy for
LADIES' AILMENTS
Is THOMASSO'S "Magic" FEMALE PILLS which are the acknowledged Leading Remedy for Correcting all Irregularities and Removing Obstruction from any cause.

These Pills are not made from Steel, Pennyroyal, Bitter Apple, or Myrrh, but from drugs far more efficacious.

Of Chemists, 1/1½ & 2/9, or post free 1/3 & 3/- from address below.

Send stamped envelope for Special Circulars and Testimonials.

Grand
REWARD.

Thousands of people of both sexes who suffered with Wrecked and Debilited Constitutions have received the Grand Reward of Perfect Recovery after using for a short time

LONGSTAFF'S Vigorating ELIXIR
which Permanently Restores those weakened by Early Indiscretions, Imparts Youthful Vigour, Restores Vitality.

The only guaranteed remedy for Impaired Memory, General Debility from overwork, and for Fagged, Weary, and Worn-out Constitutions.

Large bottle, 5/-; half-size, 3/1. Post free from address below.

DEAFNESS CURED,
Safely, Rapidly, and Permanently,
BY USING
"EROZONE,"
Which has Restored the Hearing of Thousands.
THOUSANDS OF TESTIMONIALS.
None genuine without the word "EROZONE."
1/1½ per bottle of all Chemists, or post free 1/3.

L. THOMASSO,
148, Westminster Bridge Road,
LONDON, S.E.

Leonio Thomasso's remedies. *The Ipswich Journal, Saturday 2 September 1893. Image © THE BRITISH LIBRARY BOARD. ALL RIGHTS RESERVED. Image reproduced with kind permission of the British Newspaper Archive (www.britishnewspaper-archive.co.uk)*

the subject, *The Fruits of Philosophy* by Charles Knowlton. By the 1890s, firms such as E.J. Lambert of Dalston offered a selection of devices, including the 1891 Paragon Sheath, the Sanitas Sponge with Quinine Compound and a Combined Appliance that could either be used as a condom or rolled up into a shape rather like a miniature bowler hat for covering the woman's cervix. Their catalogue also freely recommended *The Wife's Handbook*, whose author, Henry A. Allbutt, had been struck off the Medical Register in 1887 for publishing this 'obscene' work at a low enough price to be widely accessible. But promoting these products in the newspapers could prove tricky. Editors had to be careful not to risk charges of obscenity, and although contraceptives occasionally appeared in the cheaper papers such as the *Illustrated Police News*, they were not part of the proliferation of eye-catching pictorial advertisements enjoyed by consumers of other products. *The Lancet's* investigation revealed that some proprietors of female pills also dealt with 'Malthusian appliances', only promoting them to the customer once she had expressed an interest in removing an 'obstruction'. Alongside the difficulty of getting 'filthy' adverts accepted, this could reflect advertisers' recognition of a greater demand for abortifacients than for birth control devices.

The Lancet's investigations coincided with the trial of Richard, Edward and Leonard Chrimes, whose business selling 'Lady Montrose's Miraculous Female Medicinal Tabules' took an overambitious turn and resulted in the brothers' conviction for blackmail. They had posed as a public official and written to their customers, threatening imprisonment for the crime of abortion or attempted abortion. The charges would be dropped on receipt of 2 guineas.

The case revealed the huge market for abortifacients. Although most of the 12,000 women on the Chrimes' mailing list had got there by entering prize draws, almost 3,000 subsequently responded to circulars for the medicine and were frightened enough to reply to the blackmail attempt, enclosing the money or asking for time to raise it.

During her trial in 1877, Annie Besant had argued that prevention of conception warded off the greater evil of abortion: 'I hold that to destroy life, after it once lives, is the most immoral doctrine that can be put forward.' Yet, twenty years later, many women did not agree. The Chrimes case revealed that thousands of women wished to terminate pregnancy. Abortion, for them, was perhaps not a last resort but an obvious option. It did not require the insertion of an uncomfortable pessary, an embarrassing attempt to persuade an overbearing husband to pay for and wear a condom, or an inconvenient requirement to use a vaginal douche in an overcrowded house whose only water supply was that fetched by the woman herself. Perhaps more importantly, abortion was a familiar tradition, unlike the new mechanical devices. Outside the commercial world, folkloric methods of ending pregnancy had long been used by women, with herbal recipes passed on between generations and from neighbour to neighbour.

Proprietors trod on shaky ground between meeting this demand and keeping out of trouble. Even after purchase, they were careful not to be explicit about the goal of their remedies. One advised customers seeking abortion to consult a medical man. Although *The Lancet* found this 'a fairly impudent suggestion' it was nevertheless possible for women to find doctors prepared to provide this service. One of them was an associate of Thomasso, Dr James Ady, who offered a 'private hospital' – a rented flat – for the purpose.

His dealings with Ady meant that in 1897, Leonio Thomasso ended up with more to worry about than an unpaid advertising bill. The two were arrested on suspicion of providing an abortion for a 20-year-old French needlewoman,

Marguerite Barron. On searching Thomasso's rooms at 18 Featherstone Buildings, High Holborn, the police found a number of 'mischievous drugs' and Ady had allegedly used a surgical instrument. Other cases showed that this was not a one-off – evidence was given in court that two women named Jane Smith and Ada Cheek had also sought Ady and Thomasso's services. The men were found guilty and sentenced to seven years' penal servitude.

Ady's history did not serve him well in court. He had been expunged from the Medical Register in 1896 after attempting to sue the *Sun* newspaper for libel. In a sensationalist account of baby farming, murder and abortion called 'The Massacre of the Innocents', investigative journalists Isobel Priestley and Herbert Cadett interviewed a number of shady characters, including a doctor who indicated that he could arrange for an advanced pregnancy to end in stillbirth. Although he was not named, James Ady recognised himself and took the *Sun* to court, where his case was promptly thrown out.

Mr Justice Channell, who tried Ady and Thomasso at the Old Bailey in January 1898, described the pair as 'very dangerous persons'. The danger, however, lay not in the physical consequences of bungled abortions. It was a moral danger, intensified by the very fact that Thomasso and Ady were highly skilled at what they did.

Although not always with the noblest of motives, retailers like Thomasso and practitioners like Ady recognised women's desire to exert control over their own bodies, and saw the value of meeting this demand. Their perceived threat to the moral fabric of society was of more concern to the judge than the safety of patients, who were left to take their chances in less competent hands.

20

A NEW MAN AFTER ONE VIGOROUS APPLICATION

Anti-Stiff – a name contrary to the philosophy of today's email spammers – was a boon to the athletes of the 1890s. A muscle rub, it was intended to ward off aches and fatigue during sporting endeavour and its promoter claimed that 'some athletes are so fond of it that they rub it all over them'.

Unlike the messier liquid liniments that served a similar purpose, Anti-Stiff was a semi-solid substance packaged in a tin. U.S. publication the *Western Druggist* listed the product's contents as petrolatum with some essential oils and colouring – a simple but 'pleasant unguent' so convenient and portable that it soon became popular with cyclists, who could carry it en route without the worry of dropping a glass bottle or spilling it down their clothes if they stopped to use it miles from home.

Adverts for Anti-Stiff regularly appeared in *Cycling: An Illustrated Weekly*, which began publication on 24 January 1891 and soon became a hit for its attractive layout, informative articles, humorous snippets and lively writing style. Right from the first issue, Anti-Stiff had a prominent advertising presence, asking readers: 'Can you wonder that you lost that race? Why, you did not use "Anti-Stiff!"'

Testimonials abounded from the top cyclists of the day. C.A. Smith, who held the Brighton Coach Record (whereby cyclists would attempt to beat the times recorded by the old mail coaches between London and Brighton) said he was well rubbed down with Anti-Stiff before setting off on his ride. Cycling pioneer John Keen also gave an endorsement, writing that he had used every other preparation known, but found none equal to Anti-Stiff.

The product's advent coincided with a boom in cycling. From the 1880s onwards, bicycle designs became safer and easier to ride, opening up the highways to those who could not afford to travel by carriage or horseback. The mobility of women increased too and with it their physical health and independence. While unfortunate occurrences such as the death of a female cyclist after the exertions of a ride in 1894 gave critics fodder to condemn cycling as unwomanly and the 'lady cyclist' could suffer catcalls from cabbies and even physical interference with her bike or her clothing (a situation that disgracefully persists today), the freedom offered by a bicycle was too important to give up.

The *British Medical Journal* referred to beliefs that women were prone to excess in exercise, inexperienced at 'practis[ing] the careful restraint in such matters to which men are accustomed'. The *BMJ*, however, was adamant that women should 'treat all such sage advice as at least superfluous', for the benefits of cycling outweighed any risk. Support for the sorority of 'wheelwomen' also came from clerical quarters, with Canon Deane of Chichester noticing in 1902 that pubs had to become very respectable to attract their custom, and that they had a 'refining and elevating influence' on those establishments that did meet their standards. The practicalities of cycling also required adaptations to clothing, and as some female cyclists adopted knickerbocker outfits reminiscent of the Bloomerism of the 1850s, the question of 'rational dress' became ripe for campaigning on a wider scale.

The visible, active woman on a bicycle, throwing off perceived female frailty by becoming physically stronger, could be out in all weathers, travelling around without a chaperone, going where she liked, when she liked and remaining out of the house for longer periods of time. (Bearing in mind that for much of the Victorian period there was little provision of public toilets for women, limiting how long one could remain out and about.) 'Cleopatra', the female cycling columnist for *Bow Bells: A Magazine of General Art and Literature for Family Reading*, recommended Anti-Stiff as early as 1890, before the cycling craze had really taken off among women. Cleopatra, who was a fan of practical dress and referred to cycling men as 'the male things', illustrates how the lady cyclist departed from the image of Victorian womanhood. After 'ploughing through heavy mud for three hours in plenty of rain', an old sprain was playing up so she rubbed it with Anti-Stiff and got a good night's pain-free sleep. A friend of Cleopatra's, too, could 'walk miles in comfort' after using the product on a toe that she had broken as a child.

Anti-Stiff was not just for cyclists, however – it was for anyone who hoped to exhibit sporting prowess, including footballers, boxers, runners and skaters. The latter suffered from the lack of sufficiently icy surfaces all year round, making it difficult to keep in shape, so Anti-Stiff was on hand to ease the muscles gently into a new skating season, ensuring that 'the excitement may be continued when wished' rather than being cut short by aching legs.

The footballer of the 1890s might not have enjoyed the same lifestyle as his twenty-first-century counterpart, but he was invited to view Anti-Stiff as one of the finer things in life: 'An article of this kind is a real luxury, and when once it is tried by a footballer, he will always keep a tin of Anti-Stiff handy, and carry it about with him as valued as his watch.'

On his salary of £4 a week, the professional footballer could easily afford Anti-Stiff at 6*d* or 1*s* a tin, but it was

ANTI-STIFF

Is a marvellous preparation for Strengthening the Muscular System. With Anti-Stiff there is no faith required; it goes straight for the muscles, and you can feel it at work. It has a peculiarly warming, comforting, and stimulating effect on all weak or stiff muscles and sinews. Quick in its action, and cleanly and pleasant in use.

Rub it into the muscles every night for a fortnight, and you will be pleased at its supporting and strengthening properties. There is not, nor has been, anything like it till now. It differs from all Oils, Embrocations, and Liniments, both in substance and effect.

Some athletes are so fond of it that they rub it all over them.

CYCLISTS.—It was to cyclists that Anti-Stiff was first introduced, and they quickly welcomed it, as it just met a need. Cyclists required something that would be easily carried, that would prevent the dreaded stiffness resulting from over-used muscles, and a preparation that would strengthen the sinews. It was used by M. A. Holbein on his record 24 hours' ride. By the three consecutive "Brighton Record" breakers before and during those feats. By Felix Greville when training for the Hill Climbing Medal, which he obtained. By R. J. Mecredy when training for his Championships. By Harry Parsons, during the summer, when training for his records—5 to 60 miles. By E. Campbell, Royal Scottish B.C., when winning his 1890 races. By nearly every winner of races and records during 1890.

ATHLETES.—H. Griffin, Handicapper, N.C.U., Jan. 7, 1891—"Personally I can speak in very high terms of it. During 1890 I used it on several occasions, notably for a stiffened shoulder through "putting the shot," which it quickly put right "like a shot."

GYMNASTS and COMEDIANS—Brothers Harrison (two Macs) say:—"We can with pleasure testify to the remarkable preparation called Anti-Stiff, having found it matchless for stiffness consequent on our knock about business. We shall be most happy to recommend it to our brother and sister professionals."

HARRIERS.—Hon. Sec. of Spartan Harriers writes—"I have tried your Anti-Stiff, and shall certainly recommend all the members of our champion team to use it, when training for the Southern Coun-

ties' and National Cross-Country Championships, as it is a good embrocation for removing stiffness and for strengthening the muscles. Those of them that already use it speak highly of it.—G. Gardiner." (The Spartan Harriers hold the Championship of 1889 and 1890). Sid Thomas writes, December 30, 1890—"I have used Anti-Stiff several times this year, and have found it worth *all* that the proprietor claims it to be."

BOXERS use Anti-Stiff.—J. Hoare, Middle-weight Amateur Champion, 1890, writes November 22, 1890—"I have come to the conclusion that Anti-Stiff is invaluable to all boxers. Previous to my entering for the Amateur Championship this year, I found it very beneficial in strengthening the muscles of the body and promoting quickness which is essential."

SWIMMERS.—W. Evans, the 100, 220, 500 and 880 yards, and Salt Water Amateur Champion of 1890, writes December 15—"I tried Anti-Stiff on November 25, rubbing it well in, then went for a swim of a mile and a half in the Canal; to my surprise I did not feel the water cold, but came out as fresh as a lark. I will always use it in open water championships."

PEDESTRIANS—C. W. V. Clarke, ex-Amateur Walking Champion, writes Dec. 23, 1890—"I have tried your Anti-Stiff, and am only sorry I had not known of it before. I think it the most excellent strength giver and preserver I have ever tried, and that is a good many. Unless I am mistaken it will get me back to the form I showed three years ago, when I won the Championship of England and Canada."

Sold in Tins, at 6d., 1s., and 2s. 6d., by Chemists, Athletic Agents, etc., or *free by return post, with booklet containing directions, for 7 or 12 Stamps, or 2s. 6d. Postal Orders, from*

A. A. WILSON, Chemist, CHISLEHURST.

Anti-Stiff. *Author's collection*

valued enough for clubs to take responsibility for providing it. According to Charles Edwardes, who wrote on 'The New Football Mania' in 1891, Anti-Stiff was part of an expenditure that left it difficult for any club of consequence to operate for under £1,000 a year. Edwardes's amusing article implies that the referee could have done with the product on occasions too – his 'not wholly delightful' calling could see him thrown in a pond, pelted with mud or snowballs, or having his hat knocked off if he dared to appear in public after the match. (Edwardes also argued that 'A free breakfast table and football gratis' was a campaign slogan guaranteed to win votes for any political party bold enough to use it.)

Notts County coach Harry Kirk reported that his players considered Anti-Stiff 'grand stuff' and the *Blackburn Standard*'s football columnist, 'Wanderer', was a fan too:

> I do not pretend that it will produce hair on a bald head or mend on the instant a broken leg, but in cases within my knowledge it has not merely removed the stiffness of a protracted walk or an unduly long spin on the ice, but it converted one of my limping friends with an ankle big enough for two, into a new man after one vigorous application.

Field athlete H. Griffin also recommended Anti-Stiff: 'Personally, I can speak in very high terms of it. During 1890 I used it, notably for a stiffened shoulder through "putting the shot," which it quickly put right "like a shot."' I see what you did there, Mr Griffin.

Joseph Wilson, Anti-Stiff's proprietor, could attribute part of his success to his willingness to make retailers' lives easier. He appealed to chemists to carry Anti-Stiff as a product line, offering them free publicity by naming them as stockists in his adverts.

Chemists, however, were not the only outlet for Anti-Stiff. The bicycle sales and repair trade formed another obvious route to the target market, and Wilson offered to print businesses' headed paper free of charge provided he could include a discreet advert. With marketing techniques so focused on what the customer could get out of the deal, it is no surprise that Anti-Stiff soon became well-known enough to get mentions in entertainment magazines such as *Punch* and *Fun*.

In May 1891, however, the latter publication didn't give anyone much fun when it printed an Anti-Stiff joke so dire that it required a cringe-making Bruce Forsyth-style explanation of the punchline:

> It should be sold in Turkey, for there there are millions of muscle men (Mussulmen).

21

A HORSE FOR EVERY HOME

'A canter is a cure for every evil,' wrote Benjamin Disraeli. But a canter also poses the risk of a broken neck, and owning a horse involves a lot of mud and vet bills. What was the safe, sanitised alternative for the well-to-do health-conscious person of the 1890s?

Those wishing for the benefits of riding without committing to a lifetime of shit-shovelling and chilblains could invest in a Hercules Horse-Action Saddle from Messrs Vigor & Co. of 21 Baker Street. The original home exercise machine, it enabled people of all ages, shapes and sizes (at least, up to 15 stone) to enjoy trotting in the safety of their own drawing room.

The periodical *Le Follet: Journal du Grande Monde* said in May 1895:

> It is difficult to believe that any pleasure, or exercise, can in any way equal that of Riding, and to be told that an inanimate automaton, can produce equally beneficial effects on the lungs, and the internal organs, – the circulation, and the digestion, – the nerves and the figure, – sounds like a fairy tale of some 'Magic Steed'.

The main claims for the Horse-Action Saddle were that it 'rouses torpid livers, quickens the circulation, mitigates hysteria and insomnia, cures gout and rheumatism, removes general debility, creates appetite, cures dyspepsia, reduces obesity' – mostly conditions that would benefit from exercise in general. The adverts' assertions that the Saddle could trot, canter and gallop imply that it moved independently, like a genteel version of a fairground buckaroo ride, but this was not the case. The machine's concertina-like casing contained four horizontal wooden platforms separated by springs. The rider's own movements dictated the pace – an invalid could simulate a gentle walk while a more robust person could shout 'Tally ho!' and build up a furious gallop over imaginary five-bar gates. A control on the front adjusted the tension so that adventurous riders could experience a 'bone-shaker' feel, should they so wish.

Horse and Hound described the Saddle as 'a wonderful invention' that possessed 'all the elements of horse exercise, with neither the danger or expense', while the *Sporting Times* recommended it to anyone with a torpid liver, saying 'Ten minutes' gallop before breakfast will give the rider a Wiltshire labourer's appetite'.

Pamphlets featured a cartoon of a horse and rider in mid-calamity, with the slogan: 'DON'T RIDE HORSES but ride the Hercules Horse-Action Saddle.'

A description of the contraption in the *London Standard* presents it as 4 feet tall and 30 inches square. Minimal adaptions allowed it to be ridden either side-saddle or astride.

In 1895 Vigor & Co. advertised the Saddle with the strapline 'How to Enjoy Influenza', recommending the product to people confined to their rooms by indisposition. Although the idea of bouncing cheerfully through a bout of the flu seems a little far fetched, the Saddle gained doctors' approval as a wholesome form of exercise. To recreate as accurately as possible the experience of real horse exercise, the rider should open all the windows.

The Horse-Action Saddle, though primarily an aid to health, was also useful for beginner riders to improve their seat without the confusion of trying to develop a good hand at the

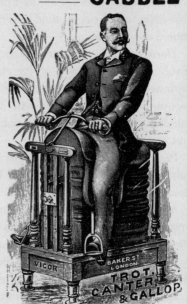

The **Readiest** *Road* **to** **Health**

Is by means of PHYSICAL EXERCISE,

and the easiest and readiest mode of Exercise is by using

VIGOR'S HORSE-ACTION

SADDLE

Which not only provides, as Dr. GEORGE FLEMING, C.C., writes, "**A PERFECT SUB-STITUTE FOR THE LIVE HORSE**" but acts so benefi-cially upon the system as to be of almost priceless value. It

PROMOTES
   GOOD SPIRITS
QUICKENS THE
   CIRCULATION,
STIMULATES
   THE LIVER
REDUCES
   CORPULENCE
CREATES
   APPETITE
CURES
   INDIGESTION
   AND GOUT.

The Field: "We have had an opportunity of trying one of the Hercules Horse-Action Saddles and found it very like that of riding on a horse; the same muscles are brought into play as when riding."

The World: "It is good for the figure, good for the complexion, and especially good for the health.

PARTICULARS AND TESTIMONIALS POST FREE.

Vigor, 21, Baker St., London.

Vigor's Horse–Action Saddle. *Author's collection*

same time. The manufacturer also recommended it for people whose disabilities – for example, visual impairment – made riding more difficult, and for those with 'mental or nervous disorders' that might affect a real horse's behaviour. Another situation that might not immediately be obvious was on a long sea journey, where the saddle could provide an alternative to tedious circuits of the deck.

The success of the Horse-Action Saddle – apparently culminating in an order from HRH the Princess of Wales, who, one would assume, had plenty of access to real horses – led to the introduction of the Vigor Home Rower, a rowing machine with a sliding seat and a counter to show the distance covered. This was said to be patronised by the Emperor of Germany, whose testimonial appeared in the adverts: 'I take exercise on the rower with sliding seat, in my Palace, every morning, and consider it a very valuable exercise.'

The foldable rowing machine was relatively portable and Messrs Vigor suggested using it when staying in hotels. At almost 56lb, it was hardly suitable for slipping into a portmanteau, but presumably its transport and assembly were for one's valet to deal with.

Vigor's premises at Baker Street included well-ventilated private rooms where people could exercise on the riding and rowing machines without the expense or commitment of buying them. This service was not, however, for all and sundry – at one guinea for eight exercises, it was clearly aimed at the comfortably off.

The evidence of newspaper classified advertisements suggests that people reconsidered their need for a Horse-Action Saddle once it began to build up a layer of dust. As early as 1894, when the Saddle had not long been on the market, second-hand examples were turning up for sale. For some, good intentions about becoming fitter had clearly ridden off into the sunset.

22

THEIR WHEELS A COMPILATION OF HUMAN BONES

In 1816, C.J. Jordan of Cannon-street-road, London, started placing ads saying he could cure 'a certain disease' (the pox) – without using mercury. He referred to himself as a surgeon but by 1818 had adopted the qualification M.D. and was calling his remedy The Cordial Balm of Rakasiri, or Nature's Infallible Restorative. His business was the East London Medical Establishment, but it might as well have been the East London Nose-Picking Establishment for all its professional credibility. With the medicine selling at 11s a bottle (33s for family size), the business was lucrative, and in August 1821 it became the Surrey and West London Medical Establishments with premises in Great Surrey Street, Blackfriars and in Berwick Street, Soho.

In early 1823, the adverts started referring to 'Drs. C. & J. Jordan'. The *Monthly Gazette of Health*, with its usual entertaining indignation, introduced the new partner as:

> Dr John Jordan, who, from the rank of distributer [*sic*] of handbills has lately been raised to the dignity of M.D. by leaping, we suppose, over a broomstick.

Balm (otherwise Balsam) of Rakasiri was, in theory, a resin from a tree species native to the Americas. It was said to have stimulant and tonic properties and had briefly been known in Britain in the early eighteenth century before its limited popularity fizzled out. The Jordans' adverts recommended their version for a variety of conditions, including consumption and scrofula, but like its inspiration, Solomon's Balm of Gilead, the main targets were venereal disease and 'nervous' disorders supposedly caused by masturbation. The natural source of the resin not being available in London, the Jordans formulated their own version – spirit of wine (rectified ethyl alcohol) flavoured with rosemary oil and sugar.

Both the *Monthly Gazette of Health* and the *Medical Adviser* campaigned against the Jordans during the 1820s and while these publications are far from objective, they make for entertaining reading. According to the *Adviser*, the Jordans had started out as pencil-sellers before taking the Cannon-street-road premises and setting up their medicine business. 'One would think to see these two fellows, standing at their door with their hands in their pockets, their hair powdered, their sleek countenance and suit of black, that they really were medical men; although to a discerning eye a peculiarly roguish cunning and an expression of innate ignorance, are labels on their front …' Of the doctors' carriage, the *Adviser* continued:

> we fancy their seat the back of an hypochondriac; their foot-board a grave-stone: their wheels a compilation of human bones; their chariot-rim decked with diseased livers; their reins the intestinal canal; their side lamps two bottles of Rakasiri; and their whip a long bill! with which the two black longtailed horses most awfully harmonize.

The *Adviser* – without much relevance, perhaps – also accused the Jordans of stealing a pig, then rather childishly printed their purported reply:

> I wont to no what you meen by tacking my karacter as you doo you rite in your book that I mede awey with a milkmans pigg but I wood

To the Afflicted with the Scurvy, Scrofula, Leprosy, Lues Venerea,

AND

Disorders originating in obstructed Perspiration, or Impurity of the Blood,

WHICH, from their having baffled the power of Professional Men, have been too rashly pronounced hopeless and incurable. There are few disorders, the cause and progress of which are so well known, and yet are treated with so little success, as the Scurvy, Leprosy, Cancer, Evil, and the like complaints, which internally sap the constitution, and outwardly disfigure the frame. The usual and most approved methods are often tried to no purpose: and a servile adherence to established practice commonly leads to the grave. As this first suggested to Drs. CHARLES and JOHN JORDAN the necessity of new experiments, so their repeated success now encourages them to offer to the Public their valuable and well-confirmed discovery. They can with full confidence affirm, that in every instance, where perseverance has been regarded, the SALUTARY DETERSIVE DROPS have ever been successful, though administered in many desperate cases of the Evil, Scurvy, and Leprosy, as well as removing pimples from the face, sore legs, or other disagreeable eruptions, and those who have unfortunately contracted a secret infection, and the bad effect of taking mercury, of drinking to excess, and of former injudicious treatment, need only make trial of the above.

Prepared only by Drs. C. & J. JORDAN, of the West London Medical Establishments, 60, Newman street, Oxford-street, and 14, Caroline-street, Bedford-square, London. In Bottles, at 11s. each; or four eleven-shilling-bottles in one family bottle for 33s., duty included, by which one 11s. bottle is saved.—The Government Label or Stamp has the words "*Charles and John Jordan, London,*" engraved on its official impression, and is uniformly pasted on the cork to protect purchasers from counterfeit imitations.

This inestimable Medicine will keep in all climates, and may be had at the Office of this Paper; and by Bacon & Kinnebrook, T. S. Buttifant, Stacy and Son, and Jarrold and Son, Norwich; C. Davie, C. Steward, and E. Markland, Yarmouth; Barker, Dereham; Finch, Swaffham; H. Paul, Fakenham; Joseph Binge, F. Prigg, and J. W. Aikin, Lynn; S. H. Blyth, North Walsham; Wm. Bane, Aylsham; F. P. Bayes, Wymondham; E. Heath, Cromer; Bishop, Eye; Cupiss, Diss; B. Priest, Lowestoft; T. Norton, and F. Mason, Beccles; W. Dyball, Bungay; C. Sewell, and J. Muskett, Harleston; Reynolds, Halesworth; G. Dunn, Saxmundham; Bird, Yoxford; G. Francis, and B. Gall, Woodbridge; F. J. Hooker, and S. B. Chapman, Ipswich; T. Pyman, Stowmarket; Dingle, and Mendham, Bury; Mrs. Stow, Hadleigh; J. W. Winter, Manningtree; T. Thompson, Harwich; Goodale, Braintree; Swinborn and Walter, Chaplin and Auston, and Holiday, Colchester; Goldsmith, Sudbury; Farrand, Clare; Rogers, Newmarket; Guy, Meggy and Chalk, Chelmsford; Nash, Whitham; Chapman, Thetford; A. J. Aikin, Maldon; and of most respectable Medicine Venders throughout the United Kingdom.

Drs. Jordan expect, when consulted by letter the usual Fee of One Pound,—addressed, Money Letter, Drs. C. & J. Jordan, West London Medical Establishment, 60, Newman-street, Oxford-street, London.—Paid double postage.

The Jordan Brothers.
Author's collection

ave you to no sir that sich like slander shall not be suffered to pass. You also say that I was a pencel pedlar this I despise and say it is a ly. I never hokd pencels I only took orders for em, and even if I did it is no affere of yours I got my bred onnestly.

To the people who had wasted money on the Balm of Rakasiri, however, the Jordans weren't such a joke. In 1828, a 'nervous young man' who had handed over more than £10 went to a magistrate and succeeded in getting his money back. During the proceedings, the Jordans threatened to make it public that he had venereal disease, but he stuck to his guns and they backed down, claiming that they were returning the money out of respect for the man's character and not because they were guilty.

Shortly afterwards, a well-to-do young woman, Miss May, consulted them for asthma and ended up £15 worse off, some of which amount she had to borrow from her sister. Finding her breathing worse and the fiery medicine affecting her stomach, she heard about the young man's success and also asked for her money back. *The Times* reported in early 1829 that:

> To this, the 'doctors' answered, that if Miss May attempted to take any such step as that young man had taken, that they would disclose the real nature of the complaint she was labouring under to her friends, which would ruin her character.

Miss May, however, was not one for giving in to bullies. Far from being shocked into silence, she said her friends knew very well she had a cough arising from asthma, and they would now also know 'the threat that you have dared to utter'. She got her lawyer, Thomas B. Cox, on the case and went to the same magistrate who had ordered the young man's refund. He told her to apply to the Middlesex Sessions for a bill of indictment for fraud. This was refused and the Jordans' lawyer, Mr Adolphus, published a notice in the *Morning Chronicle* titled

'Base and Malicious Charge of Fraud Refuted'. Purportedly
a news story about the Jordans and Mr Adolphus attending
Marlborough Street Police Court to complain against Miss
May's allegations, it described her and her lawyer as 'infamous
calumniators' trying to extort money. Mr Adolphus said:

> Who ever heard of a person making a purchase, using the article so
> purchased and then, forsooth, demanding their money back, much
> less make a charge of fraud against the tradesman so refusing? The
> attempted fraud was on their own side, and a gross attempt it was.

The doctors challenged their accusers to 'come forward and
repeat their base and unfounded charge'. To their horror,
however, Miss May was only too ready to do so. When Cox
wrote to them inviting them to appear before the magistrates
for that very purpose, they had to wriggle out of it by insisting
that they would only go if summoned by the court. They did
not turn up at the appointed time. Mr Cox was professionally
disgusted:

> Was it not monstrous, that such imposters as these men, who were
> literally a pest in society, and the direct enemies of the human race,
> should be rolling in their carriages and wallowing in wealth, while
> men of high education, who had laboriously, and at great expense,
> studied their profession and made themselves masters of medical
> knowledge, were living, in many instances, in obscurity, and scarcely
> able to supply the means of living respectably?

The more cynical among us might be tempted to say 'welcome
to real life, Mr Cox', but as the doctors realised that Miss May
was quite prepared to take them to the cleaners, they got
nervous ('Notwithstanding the anti-nervous powers of their
medicine,' commented the *Monthly Gazette of Health*). They
settled out of court, refunding Miss May's money, paying her

legal expenses and giving her £100 compensation. They also published a notice in the papers saying that their assertions in the 'Base and Malicious ...' article had no foundation, and that they expressed their 'deep regret' for having published them.

It would be nice to finish with the *Gazette's* conclusion:

> To Miss May, for her heroic conduct, and Mr. Cox, her solicitor, for the firmness with which he conducted the proceedings, the thanks of the public are due. They have completely knocked up the Balsam of Rakasira [*sic*] trade, than which a more infamous traffic has not been carried on in the most barbarous country.

But for all the *Gazette's* confidence, the Jordans' business was far from knocked up. For a while, they focused on a new product – the Salutary Detersive Drops, aimed at those suffering from scrofula and venereal disease. These afflictions they put down to the 'intemperance and luxury of the age'. Patients weak enough to destroy their own constitutions through a love of sensual gratification could recover sufficiently even to gain mastery over the weather: 'Hail, rain or snow can be no obstacle to any person taking this medicine.'

Briefly in 1833, the Jordans' West London Medical Establishment at 60 Newman Street off Oxford Street became the 'London College of Health' in imitation of the famous Hygeist, James Morison, whose British College of Health at King's Cross was doing a roaring trade in Vegetable Pills. With Charles as President and John as Vice-President, the London College advertised its belief that 'all diseases originate from a diseased condition of the blood, and that the medicines which are likely to effect a certain cure of every disease, must derive their origin from the vegetable creation'.

This was the basis of Morison's Hygeian theory, yet the Jordans were no mere disciples. Audaciously, they claimed to be the philosophy's original advocates. The Balm of Rakasiri and the Salutary Detersive Drops were joined by Jordan's Vegetable Pills as components of a three-part system called the 'Vegetable Universal Medicines'. To the casual newspaper reader, the Jordans' lengthy advertisements promising cures for everything from cholera to the decay consequent upon masturbation were barely distinguishable from Morison's. Even the format and dose of the Vegetable Pills was the same, with two strengths, Nos 1 and 2, to be taken in quantities of up to twenty at a time.

The London College's existence was brief and by the end of 1833 the Balm of Rakasiri was once again the main product, focusing on invigorating the decayed juices of those who had got up to imprudence in youth. The Jordans also began to spread their net wider than the metropolis, setting up a branch in Leeds.

Around 1840, they dropped the M.D. qualification and became Messrs Jordan and Co., Surgeons, with premises in Bristol too. Later that decade, a medicine called Balm of Rakasiri was being sold by Messrs Henry & Co., Liverpool, with a very similar advertising style to the Jordans, and in the 1850s Messrs Lewis were the proprietors. The name finally changed to Dr Lucas and the remedy was still burning oesophagi at the end of the 1860s.

23

ITS POWER TO ASSUAGE MATERNAL PAIN

Twenty-year-old lace worker Mary Colton had tried many times to stop giving her baby the opium-based Godfrey's Cordial, but found that she could not, 'for if she did, she should not have anything to eat'.

Interruption of her low-paid work could have meant starvation, and drugging her child was the only thing that staved off this fate. Her dilemma, and that of countless other mothers in the mid-nineteenth century, became a focus of concern among those who had never experienced such poverty. Political and journalistic investigation and debate, incorporating evidence from physicians and druggists, presented the use of opiate 'soothing syrups' as an example of a 'moral cause' of disease and an explanation for high infant mortality. But underlying the concern for child welfare simmered a deeper anxiety – if a women was at work and allegedly neglecting her children, she was probably not looking after her husband very well either.

Godfrey's Cordial, along with other opiate 'soothing syrups', was ubiquitously available in Victorian Britain. Accessible even to the poorest members of society, it was cheap, addictive, dangerous and effective.

The practice of using soothing syrups for babies and toddlers attracted political attention at regular intervals throughout the century, but came to particular prominence during the 1840s, when a series of commissions on public health issues highlighted the pernicious effects of opium on working-class children's health. Yet opium products remained widely available well beyond the Pharmacy Act of 1868, which would have been the perfect opportunity to restrict their sale. In the criticism of working-class opiate use, there were more agendas at stake than the welfare of children.

The notion of the mother as a serene, self-sacrificial figure, consumed by the desire to nurture her children, had been gaining currency since the late eighteenth century. By the beginning of the Victorian period, the middle-class ideology of motherhood was shaped by the notion that the maternal feeling was intense and instinctive, a vocation that could not be replaced by another's care. The *British Mother's Journal* captured the angelic stereotype with its reminder to readers that they had been ordained by God as the guardians of His children:

> Stirred with a thrilling sense of a sacred trust reposed in her, serenely conscious of the honour with which God has crowned her, animated with the bright visions of the future, she lives above the ills and disquietudes of her condition.

And yet this selfless repose was very far from the image – and the reality – of the mother that emerged from the evidence of the Select Committees investigating the public health of manufacturing communities in the mid-nineteenth century. For public commentators viewing the working-class mother through this lens, the use of opiate 'soothers' was a direct contradiction of this vocation, because its only perceived purpose was to reduce the child's demands on its mother.

Commissions such as the Children's Employment Commission of 1842–43 and that on the State of Large Towns in 1845 were established to gather information on health issues and working conditions. Emerging from these sources is a recurring theme – that of the almost universal use of narcotic products such as Godfrey's Cordial, Dalby's Carminative, Mrs Winslow's Soothing Syrup and Atkinson's Royal Infants' Preservative. Underlying the discussion of this practice were certain assumptions about motherhood and women's work, criticising the departure of women from their sacred function and implying that the root cause of poverty was the female worker's separation from her natural role as a mother.

Throughout the commissioners' reports, the most commonly cited reason given for opium use is along the lines that it was 'in no way connected with any medical treatment; it is simply to still the infant in order that the mother may work'. Motherhood was considered such a powerful, spontaneous and natural force that *Trewman's Exeter Flying Post* could ask:

> What would society become but for the sweet influences upon it of motherhood, that thrice blessed and divine institution which more or less closely links every one's first thoughts and latest recollections with the purity and gentleness and self-denial and unquenchableness of woman's love?

This could support only one conclusion – that mothers alone were suited to looking after their children. Drugging a child in order to be able to work at an occupation for which Providence had not suited her was a desertion of this natural function. During the debate on the Factories Bill in 1844, Lord Ashley, later Earl of Shaftesbury, took a particularly strident position against women's work, using the example of the use of Godfrey's Cordial to support the argument that 'It is most desirable that mothers should not be, if possible, abstracted from their attention to their helpless infants'.

The admirable philanthropic achievements of Lord Ashley's career cannot be dismissed, but his views on infant cordials seem

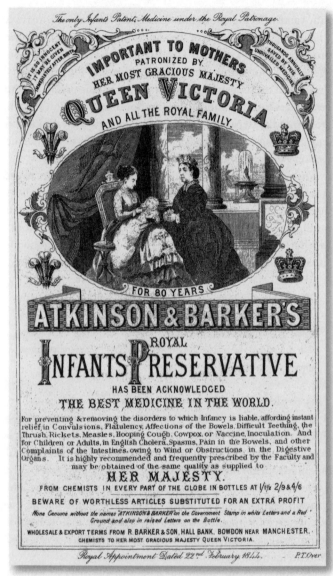

Atkinson and Barker's Royal Infants Preservative. *Image © Bodleian Library,*
University of Oxford 2008: John Johnson Collection, Food 12 (46). Copyright ©
2008 ProQuest LLC. All rights reserved

to have root in the concern that when working-class women work, working-class men are deprived of their own domestic staff: 'everything runs to waste; the house and children are deserted; the wife can do nothing for her husband and family; she can neither cook, wash, repair clothes, or take charge of the infants …'

Lord Ashley's anxieties were transparent enough to be recognised by his opponents. In reply, Sir James Graham stated, 'I will not say I thought there was exaggeration …', but the noble Lord appeared to be advocating for an end to the employment of women and children altogether, rather than a reduction of their working hours.

By this time Godfrey's Cordial, which had been around since the mid-eighteenth century, had become a generic product. Chemists made up their own versions of 'Godfrey' to their preferred formulae, and a bottle from one shop could be stronger than the one from round the corner – there was no way for the parent to know. The strength could even vary within the bottle as the opium gathered at the bottom.

Mothers were not the only people criticised for using opiate products on infants. The figure of the nurse, too, emerged as a scapegoat that deflected attention from the low wages and terrible working conditions that were leaving families struggling to survive. Day nurses, rather than mothers, bore the main responsibility for drugging children, according to Henry Mayhew's journalistic investigation into the state of labour and the poor for the *Morning Chronicle* in 1849–50. His analysis reveals attitudes among physicians and druggists that, while criticising opiate use, served to perpetuate the conditions that made it necessary. John Greg Harrison, a factory medical inspector, ascribed high infant mortality in cotton towns to drugging and poor nursing, not to 'any fatal effect inherent in factory labour'.

A recurring descriptor of nurses in the opinions of politicians and journalists is 'superannuated', presenting these older women as past any useful function. The term appears in Mayhew's article, in J.R. Coulthart's contribution to the report on the State of Large Towns, and in 'Protected Cradles', a piece by William Blanchard Jerrold in Dickens' *Household Words* in 1850. According to Jerrold, the 'ignorant nurse, redolent of laudanum', drugged children in order to be able to look after a large number of them at once. While he acknowledged the contribution of poor sanitation and malnutrition to the high rates of infant mortality in the manufacturing towns, ultimately these were 'of minor importance when taken in relation to the streams of laudanum and aniseed that stupefy their childhood'. As with the political comment of the 1840s, it was easy to blame opiates and the 'crones' who administered them than to address the issues that left those living in poverty with no other choice.

Some child minders were girls only a few years older than their charges. Their evidence to the Commissions about buying Godfrey's Cordial for those in their care and taking 'a little of it herself sometimes, because its [*sic*] nice' has a poignant aura of lost innocence.

The older nurse, however, is a more sinister figure. Like sick-nurses, midwives and monthly nurses of the Sairey Gamp ilk, the day nurse fitted into a convenient caricature of incompetence and immorality. Just as midwives' knowledge had traditionally been associated with superstition and even witchcraft in order to undermine them, the day nurse was portrayed as an 'ignorant beldam' – her age and ugliness apparently proof enough of her unsuitability.

Coming under particular scrutiny in 1871, with the Select Committee for the Protection of Infant Life, the child minder was revealed as someone 'unfit for other employment', an elderly woman who was 'very incompetent and very ignorant'. Manchester surgeon Mr W. Whitehead estimated that a huge number of women were undertaking the task, with a correspondingly high prevalence of opiate use.

The caricatured image of the 'beldam' sometimes bordered on the grotesque. In an opinion piece on the absence of a suitable crèche system, *Lloyd's Weekly Newspaper* cited the alleged case of an 'old woman, 73 years of age' placing an infant in a pot of boiling water to punish it. The story evokes the image of a witch at her cauldron and constructs a sensationalist scapegoat that ignores the economic and social reasons why a mother might have no choice but to leave her child in the care of such a person.

Through the stereotype of the 'ignorant beldam', the day nurse became a caricatured hybrid of witch and baby farmer that supported the argument that children should only be cared for by their mothers and the only means of bringing this about was for those mothers to stay at home.

Druggists, meanwhile, against the backdrop of the drive for professionalisation, also sought to confer individual responsibility for high opiate use on child minders. Mayhew found them reluctant to give evidence, but those who did respond were critical of the practice of drugging and thought that 'nurses were chiefly to blame'. As the State of Large Towns Commission recognised in 1845, the druggists were reluctant to accept their own role in the prevalence of opium use, or to lose the considerable income it raised:

> The druggists who give this evidence are respectable men – in all common dealings of life, humane men, – but custom has rendered them indifferent to the fearful consequences arising from this practice. They are not ignorant of the great details, but they have been accustomed to view them with a business eye.

The attitude was later to influence opium's place on the schedules of the Pharmacy Act in 1868, which while regulating the sale of opium preparations so that only qualified pharmacists could dispense them, did not cover patent medicines like Atkinson and Barker's Royal Infants' Preservative.

This preparation boasted the ultimate celebrity endorsement – that of Queen Victoria herself. Atkinson and Barker were 'Chemists to Her Majesty in Manchester', but quite how often she popped into their Bowdon warehouse, it is difficult to ascertain. The relationship mainly involved the company trumpeting the royal connection and assuring lowlier customers that they would receive the same quality Preservative that was sent to the Queen.

Advertising for the Royal Preservative highlights an issue that contemporary commentators largely ignored – that of the perceived beneficial effects of such products. In direct contrast to the views of political and journalistic commentators, it

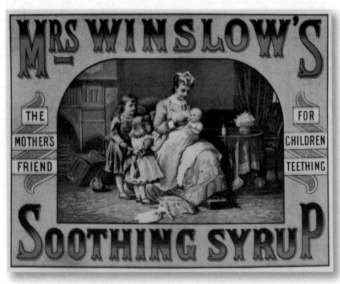

Mrs Winslow's Soothing Syrup. *Author's collection*

presented the medicine as an important part of fulfilling the ideal of motherhood:

> whether this medicine enters the palace or the cottage, the proprietor feels an honest conviction of its power to assuage maternal pain for infant suffering – to convert that pain into gladness, that suffering into balmy repose.

Advertisements contained testimonials from doctors, such as Edward Williams, described as an 'eminent physician', who considered it 'a most desirable medicine in every affection to which infants are liable'.

The original version of Godfrey's Cordial, by this time under the proprietorship of Benjamin Godfrey Windus, also emphasised the health-giving properties and appealed to parental anxiety. Windus promoted it for all ages and claimed that it had the satisfying result of assuaging 'the torment and griping of the stomach and bowels, and, by breaking off the wind, never fails to give immediate relief', but children's ailments were of particular concern. Colic and other distressing conditions could prove fatal, warned its handbills, but even if the child were to survive:

> it remains a sickly subject, and the fond hope of seeing a fine robust and spirited offspring, is at all events delayed for years, and perhaps denied for life. In ninety-nine cases out of every hundred this valuable cordial would prevent so unfortunate a result.

Judging by the language of the advertisements, it would have been neglectful *not* to have administered opiates to babies.

Mary Colton, the young woman with whom this chapter began, was advised by others in her community to give her sickly four-month-old child laudanum to 'bring it on', as the substance was thought to help babies to thrive. Her use of Godfrey and laudanum was not only to keep her daughter placid, but because traditional attitudes suggested this was the best thing for the child. Working-class mothers' motives were not necessarily as mercenary and unnatural as Lord Ashley liked to think.

The reality was, however, that opiate preparations were frequently implicated in babies' deaths. News reports of inquests carried world-weary titles such as 'Godfrey's Cordial Again' and 'Another Victim to Godfrey's Cordial'. 'Another child has been destroyed at Liverpool by a dose of Godfrey's Cordial,' lamented the *Leeds Times* in 1859, 'Will parents and nurses never learn wisdom?'

Atkinson and Barker's product, too, was still proving fatal eighteen years after the Pharmacy Act. In 1886, an inquest on the body of a six-week-old baby decided that a mere six drops of Royal Infants' Preservative had been enough to kill it, as it was already weakened by illness. Surgeon Mr H.S. Leigh told the jury that when he saw the baby the morning after the dose, 'its pupils were contracted to the size of a pin's head; it was covered with a cold, clammy sweat; it was breathing about six in the minute, and was apparently moribund'. The child 'lingered on till evening, when it died'. The mixture's composition was listed in the *Druggist's General Receipt Book* in 1878 as 6 drachms of carbonate of magnesia, 2oz of white sugar, 20 drops of aniseed oil, 2 drachms of spirit of sal volatile, 1 drachm of laudanum, 1oz of syrup of saffron, made up to a pint with caraway water. The amount of laudanum was small, but then so were the people who received it.

It was hardly surprising, however, that people believed the Preservative to be beneficial. The immediate experience of seeing a distressed baby calming down counted for a lot – and then there was the apparent official sanction for the product.

In 1876, Kilburn doctor William H. Platt wrote to the medical journals to highlight an issue he had discovered quite by accident. Local parents were finding flyers for the Royal Infants' Preservative enclosed with their children's vaccination papers. Vaccination against smallpox was compulsory and these official documents were sent out to all who had registered a birth. Platt surmised that someone from Atkinson and Barker had done a deal with the Board of Guardians to come up with this plan.

The result, he believed, was 'to induce the people receiving these papers, many of them poor and ignorant, to believe that these so-called infant preservatives are recommended by the same authority which enforces vaccination'.

With authorities like that, impoverished mothers can hardly be blamed for thinking infant soothers were a good thing.

24

THE PLAINS ARE BOUNTIFUL IN BULBS

Between March 1852 and September 1853, monthly instalments of Charles Dickens's *Bleak House* tempted readers with their eye-catching illustrated covers and affordable price of 1s. Within these covers, the 'Bleak House Advertiser' promoted commercial products, from new publications to false teeth, and from wigs to bedsteads. Inserted in part fourteen, however, after chapters 43 to 46, was an eight-page advertisement containing a narrative creation of its own.

Ali Ahmed's Treasures of the Desert were a set of three remedies whose proprietor created an aura of exoticism, presenting them as traditional and natural alternatives to harsh western medicine. The range comprised the Sphairopeptic Pill for liver and digestive complaints, the Pectoral Antiphthisis Pill to fight off colds, asthma and consumption and the Antiseptic Malagma – a plaster for use on ulcers, wounds, gangrene and varicose veins. With a month to wait until the next instalment of *Bleak House*, an advertising insert stood a good chance of being read, and by using an engaging story rather than a hard sell, the proprietor had the opportunity to get the reader on side.

The pamphlet drew the reader in with an unexpectedly up-front reference to quackery: 'WHAT! more atrocities in the quack line? More conspiracies against the poor stomach? Such we can easily believe to be the exclamation of the reader as he scans the heading of this paper.' Scepticism is all very well when you're in fine fettle, however. The pamphlet went on to remind the reader that health problems could be lurking round the next corner. He or she would be prudent to keep these remedies in mind.

Ali Ahmed Mascuieli was said to have been a medieval Persian physician, exiled for political reasons from the land of his birth and, after a requisite period of wandering in the desert, settling at Aleppo in Syria. A doctor of great erudition and humanity, he published a book on the composition of medicine from vegetable matter – a work that was sadly not available to the Victorian reader, for all but one of its copies had been destroyed by order of a tyrannical and ignorant Caliph.

On his deathbed, Ali Ahmed confided the recipes to his relatives, who handed them down through the generations until, in the nineteenth century, they attracted the attention of 'an excellent and philanthropic Englishman' who saw it as his duty to share them with the world. The pamphlet used a decorative border and examples of calligraphy (described by Bernard Darwin in his 1930 book *The Dickens Advertiser* as 'lovely Arabic curly-wiggles'!) to emphasise the long tradition of eastern medicine from which the remedies had sprung.

After a brief introduction, the pamphlet featured a letter from a friend of the proprietor in Damascus, who had reintroduced the remedies there to the fury of the resident European physicians. The letter writer becomes a character in the pamphlet's narrative, entertaining the reader with the tale of a particularly incompetent doctor:

one idiot actually went so far as to say, that he would complain of me to the local authorities for practising without a licence – a threat I very soon silenced by recalling to his mind the ludicrous fact of his having ordered a wholesale supply of common table-salt, believing that it was some cheap but valuable medicine (from its being invoiced under

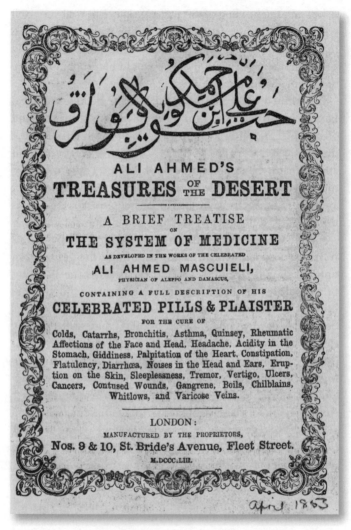

Ali Ahmed's Treasures of the Desert. *Image © Bodleian Library, University of Oxford 2008: John Johnson Collection, Patent Medicines 1 (6a). Copyright © 2008 ProQuest LLC. All rights reserved*

its scientific name), which would answer his ends to dose the poor
natives with.

In contrast to such scientific fecklessness, the letter-writer lauds
'the simple native physician', whose drugs are 'the kindest gifts
of nature to suffering humanity'. Unlike the violent substances
such as strychnine and morphine prescribed by European
doctors, the eastern practitioner's drugs were 'simple and pure;
the mountainside furnishes him with herbs and roots, and
the plains are bountiful in bulbs'. The notions that a remedy
stems from ancient, traditional knowledge, that it is safe and
natural, and that narrow-minded orthodox doctors hate it are
all, of course, to be found in dubious advertising today. Punch
pointed out that the medicines would probably work if taken
as part of the lifestyle enjoyed by Ali Ahmed. Together with a
sparse diet, nothing but water to drink, and plenty of galloping
through the desert, they would no doubt remove 'the worst
congestion of the liver that ever affected alderman'.

So, just how exotic were these medicines? *Cooley's
Cyclopaedia of Practical Receipts, Processes, and Collateral
Information in the Arts, Manufactures, Professions and Trades,
including Medicine, Pharmacy and Domestic Economy* (Fourth
Edition, 1864) gave the ingredients: The Antiseptic Malagma
comprised lead plaster, gum thus (frankincense or, more
likely, thickened turpentine), salad oil and beeswax, spread
onto calico. The Pectoral Pill, which adverts claimed
'never causes that nausea invariably connected with cough
medicines, where Ipecacuanha and other baneful drugs are
commonly used', contained myrrh, squills, white soft soap,
aniseed oil, treacle – and ipecacuanha. The Sphairopeptic
Pills were aloes, colocynth pulp, rhubarb, myrrh, scammony,
ipecacuanha, cardamom seeds, soft soap, oil of juniper and
treacle. The advertising also stated that the pills were 'silver-
gilt in the Oriental style', to neutralise any unpleasant taste,

a practice traditionally thought to have originated with the tenth-century Persian physician, Avicenna.

The influence of Ali Ahmed's medicines stretched even further east with the claim that they had cured Prince Chou Faa of Siam of a bad cough, 'which not all the skill of the resident American physicians could cure or even alleviate'. Two doses of the Pectoral Pills did the trick and inspired Prince Chou Faa to distribute them among all Bangkok's doctors.

Appropriately for the advert's placement in *Bleak House*, Prince Chou Faa was said to be a Dickens fan. In 1852, the year before Ali Ahmed's medicines rose to prominence, Frederick Arthur Neale's *Narrative of a Residence at the Capital of the Kingdom of Siam* described him as a keen scholar of English and a 'perfect gentleman' who indulged in a hearty chuckle over *The Pickwick Papers*.

It is not recorded whether he became equally engrossed in the story of Lady Dedlock and Esther Summerson, but if he did, perhaps he would have been amused at the sight of his name in their company.

25

NO ONE COULD SUPPOSE
HE MEANT ANY HARM

When you're under the weather and you Google your symptoms in an attempt to convince yourself that you are about to die, spare a thought for Jean Landess, whose perusal of *Chambers's Encyclopaedia* was the beginning of a tragic chain of events.

In May 1868, 39-year-old Mrs Landess, of Paisley, had just weaned her youngest child and had developed what she called a 'weed' in her right breast. She sought medical help, and the family doctor lanced and poulticed two small abscesses.

Mrs Landess, however, discovered from the *Encyclopaedia* that the needle-like pains she was experiencing were a symptom of breast cancer. On the recommendation of an acquaintance, she sent for Aberdeen cancer-doctor Alexander Paterson, who had built up a strong reputation as a healer over the past twenty years and happened to be temporarily residing in Glasgow.

Paterson was a former shoemaker who had added the treatment of cancer and sprains to a repertoire of talents that included not only cobbling but also literary endeavour – in 1839 he had published a song called *Piper Tam and the Priest of Methlic*. So popular did he become that he gave up his successful shoemaking business in about 1853 and devoted his time to travelling around Scotland by invitation from people with cancer. While not actively claiming to have any medical qualifications, and advertising as 'Mr Paterson', he went about his practice without 'by any means objecting to the title of "Dr." in a general way'.

During the 1860s, he represented himself as head of the 'Cancer Institution' in George Street, Aberdeen, announcing his availability for consultation by means of notices in the local papers of each town he visited. In September 1865, for example, he saw patients at Elgin, Dufftown and Lossiemouth, moving down to Dundee in October. On one occasion, his reputation even took him as far as Florence, where he attended a Hungarian 'lady of position'. Sadly, he could not save her, but was financially rewarded for his efforts.

Paterson told Mrs Landess that she did have cancer, but not to worry – it could easily be removed. The first stage of the treatment was a fly-blister (a plaster of cantharides) that would take off the surface of the skin, leaving it ready to absorb his cancer-curing salve. After the plaster had been on for about twelve hours, he applied a calico dressing smeared with ointment and instructed the patient to renew it every day.

The ointment caused a severe burning pain in Mrs Landess's breast. She developed a violent headache, thirst, vomiting, numbness in her limbs, loss of appetite and sleeplessness. By Paterson's next visit on 25 May, most of the tissue covered by the ointment had turned black, but he saw this as a good thing and reassured Mrs Landess that the treatment was going well. Shortly after he left, however, the pain became intolerable and Mrs Landess felt faint. The inflammation in the breast was creeping up into her right shoulder and arm, and by the next day pains were shooting through her belly. Never, she said, could she survive such another night's suffering.

A mustard plaster on her abdomen and a poultice on her breast made her feel more comfortable, but on 27 May she had a fit. Her husband Robert described her appearance as 'being like a "half-felled cow". Foam issued from her mouth, and she roared most unnaturally.'

On recovering consciousness, she said that she had 'been in a queer place, that she felt, as it were, a dart go through her, that she then became insensible, and had no further recollection of what happened to her during the fit'. Later that afternoon she felt better than she had done since the start of the treatment and was able to eat, but between nine and ten o'clock she suddenly said, 'There it is again,' fell into another fit and died.

Douglas Maclagan, Professor of Medical Jurisprudence at Edinburgh University, carried out a post-mortem examination and confirmed that Mrs Landess had never had breast cancer. There were traces of arsenic in her organs and when he analysed Paterson's salve he discovered that it was 49 per cent arsenic and 51 per cent lard.

The Medical Act of 1858 legislated for the registration of qualified practitioners but did not ban the unqualified from practising. When Paterson was brought to trial charged with culpable homicide, the question was not whether he should have been allowed to attend Mrs Landess in the first place, but whether he had been negligent when administering a dangerous medicine. According to Paterson's defence, Mrs Landess asked for his help in the full knowledge that he was an unregistered practitioner. Several witnesses came forward to say that he had cured them.

The judge, Lord Ardmillan, must have been in a particularly good mood that day. In summing up, he advised the jury not to be too swayed by the fact that Paterson was unqualified, but to take into account his experience, the apparent cures of the witnesses and the fact that any medical man could muck up sometimes. 'A mere mistake,' he said, 'did not imply culpability.'

The jury found Paterson guilty. Lord Ardmillan, however, told him that 'no one could suppose he meant any harm to the unfortunate woman Landess' and sent him to prison for just four months. Paterson took the sentence with good humour, remarking after his release that 'if all the M.D.s had the same measure meted out to them for professional work, the jails of the country would be crammed with doctors like as many hospitals!'

In the 1850s the issue of cancer-doctors had attracted the attention of Thomas Spencer Wells, later to become surgeon to the royal family, who published his 'Cancer Cures and Cancer Curers' in 1860.

'It is a singular fact,' Wells wrote, 'that we are never without some fashionable "cancer-curer".' He was referring to a number of expensive practitioners operating in London and on the continent, including M. Vriès, the 'Black Doctor', whose positive outlook in even the worst cases could not keep him out of prison in Paris. In England, an American cancer specialist, J. Weldon Fell, was charging 100 guineas for removing tumours with a salve containing bloodroot and the caustic zinc chloride.

But as Wells acknowledged, whether a cancer patient went to top surgeons, paid a fortune for corrosive salves or called in a local healer, the odds were still against them. He was not surprised that cancer-curers were so popular, for they offered

---

C A N C E R, &c.

MR PATERSON, of the Cancer Institution, No 196 GEORGE STREET, Aberdeen, intends paying a PROFESSIONAL VISIT (by invitation), to ELGIN and its neighbourhood, when he proposes to arrive on 4th SEPTEMBER next, for the treatment of CANCER and UL- CERATED, and other Chronic and malignant Diseases, and, during his stay, he will visit DUFFTOWN and LOSSIE- MOUTH.

In the meantime, communications from parties desir- ing his services, may be addressed to the care of Mr PETER MURRAY, Hopeman, or to Mr CUMMING, No 16 Guildry Street, Elgin.

Aberdeen, 21st August, 1865.

Alexander Paterson. *Elgin Courier, Friday 1 September 1865. Image*

something the medical profession had neglected – hope. Doctors might have felt they were being honest when they considered a case incurable, but these bleak prognostications effectively meant washing one's hands of the patient and waving them off on a quest for a miracle.

'Cancer-curers', meanwhile, were prepared to offer hope in abundance. Paterson, for example, had reassured Mrs Landess that her supposed cancer would be simple to remove because it was not hard at the back. When her breast turned black, he was quick to say that this meant it was 'doing very well'. M.Vriès in Paris made a career of his ability to 'cheer his victim on to the last, enabling him, as it were, to die easy'.

Wells chastised his medical readers for guiding patients into the hands of empirics by neglecting simple measures to relieve suffering even where a cure was impossible. He cited the case of a lady with a severely ulcerated tumour of the breast:

> The odour of her room, and indeed of the whole house, was so overpowering that the comfort of the inmates was destroyed; servants could not be kept and even nurses could only be induced to stay by high wages and an almost unlimited allowance of brandy.

Chloride of zinc, administered by Dr Fell, had a corrosive effect on the wound but it was also deodorising, relieving at least a little of the woman's distress during her last few months.

Fear of surgery was another reason for seeking out alternative treatment. Although chloroform was in widespread use by the time Wells was writing, this did not mean people would leap confidently onto the operating table without a care in the world. By exaggerating the dangers and pain of surgery, cancer-curers could make their own methods appear the more attractive option. In 1856, Dr Fell convinced the Christian writer and landscape painter Emily Gosse that his treatment left only a 20 per cent risk of recurrence of the disease, compared to 80 per cent recurrence in patients undergoing surgery.

Assured that treatment by salve was also less painful than an operation, Mrs Gosse went under his care, the agony of which is described in horrifying detail in *A Memorial of the Last Days on Earth of Emily Gosse* by her husband Philip Henry Gosse. When the ointment alone did not heal the tumour, Dr Fell offered to extract it, blistering the skin with nitric acid and then scarifying the tumour's surface in order to help it absorb the 'purple mucilaginous substance' that would destroy the tissue. After four weeks of pain so intense that Emily could neither 'lie, sit or stand', the tumour was ready to be removed, and Dr Fell used a ring of corrosive plaster around its edges in order to detach it from the flesh – a process that took another two weeks.

A furrow, gradually deepening, formed between the living flesh and the hard and black tumour, and this was filled with pus. The sensation now became that of a heavy weight dragging at the breast, and this feeling increased as the connexion between the parts daily diminished. At length, on Sunday, the 23rd of November, to our delight, the great insensible tumour fell out of its cavity, hanging only by a slender thread, which presently yielded, and the breast was relieved of its load – the dead body that it had so long carried about.

The delight, however, was transient. It became apparent that some malignant tissue remained in the cavity and Emily underwent the whole lengthy process a second time. Dr Fell then admitted that a third and fourth round of treatment would be necessary. Emily could not face going through it again and returned home, dying in February 1857.

The theories of cancer presented by fringe practitioners appeared logical and convincing. According to Wells, they spoke of the 'roots' of a tumour, which must be removed altogether if the disease were not to recur. They showed patients examples of preserved tumours exhibiting shreds of the surrounding tissue, lending weight to the idea that the cancer wound its insidious tendrils deep into the flesh. The orthodox method of chopping it out would leave these roots ready, like those of a pernicious weed, to send forth shoots again.

Wells himself advocated good food, pure country air, extreme cleanliness of person, sufficient exercise, clothing that did not press on the affected part, mental occupation and amusement. He also, however, suggested that bromide of potassium with cod liver oil would reduce the size of a tumour – a remedy that could just as easily have been thought up by an unqualified person.

The unfortunate fact was that if you had an aggressive malignant tumour, you were a goner, no matter whom you consulted.

Alexander Paterson continued his practice until near the end of his life, taking his skills to Belfast in 1872 when he was 62 years old. When he became ill with liver disease and its consequent dropsy, letters were still arriving with the cries for help of suffering people and 'he was so eager to do what he could, that latterly these applications had to be kept out of his ken'. He died in August 1874. Thomas Spencer Wells urged doctors never to give up seeking a cure for the terrible disease:

> We have found a specific for ague; we have found a specific for itch; we can certainly cure some forms of syphilis by iodide of potassium, and others by mercury; we can prevent small-pox by vaccination. Let us hope that the day may come when we shall possess equal power over those mysterious aberrations in the processes of nutrition and decay which lead to the deposits or formations known as tubercle and cancer.

Until that day, well-meaning incompetents and criminal fraudsters would always be on hand to offer hope.

SOURCES

1   A poisonous nostrum in one hand and the Holy Bible in the other

'Annals of Quackery', *The Medical Adviser, and Guide to Health and Long Life*, No. 17, 27 March 1824, pp. 267–271.

Cooper, Bransby Blake, *The Life of Sir Astley Cooper, Bart., interspersed with sketches from his note-books of distinguished contemporary characters*, Vol. II, John W. Parker, London, 1843.

Crell, A. F., and Wallace, W. M., *The Family Oracle of Health: Economy, Medicine, and Good Living*, J. Walker, London, 6th edition, 1824.

'Dr. Gardner's Last and Best Bedroom', *The Medical Adviser, and Guide to Health and Long Life*, No. 13, 28 February 1824, pp. 206–207.

'Dr. Gardner's Museums (Long Acre and Shoreditch High Street)', Advertising handbill, *c.* 1800, *Drug advertising ephemera: Pre-1850. Box 1*, Wellcome Library.

'Dr Gardner's Worm Medicine', *The London Medical and Surgical Spectator: Or, Monthly Register of Medicine*, Vol. 2, No. 9, April 1809.

'Dr Gardner's Worm Medicine', *The Medical Observer*, No. 1, 1806, pp. 66–72.

McCoy North, Eric, *Early Methodist Philanthropy*, The
    Methodist Book Concern, New York and Cincinnati,
    1914.

'Modern Eccentrics', *Temple Bar, A London Magazine for Town
    and Country Readers*, Vol. 17, July 1866.

Marriott, Thomas, 'Methodism in Former Days',
    The Wesleyan-Methodist Magazine, Vol. 1, July 1845,
    pp. 661–668.

Smallfield, G. (Ed.), *The Monthly Repository of Theology and
    General Literature*, Vol. XIV, London, 1819.

2   Witchcraft and such like tomfoolery

'Extraordinary Quackery and Superstition at Hull', *The Hull
    Packet and East Riding Times*, 7 June 1844, p. 5.

'Hull Midsummer General Quarter Sessions: The Case of the
    Quack Doctors', *The Hull Packet and East Riding Times*,
    5 July 1844, p. 6.

'Progress of Quackery at Hull', *The Hull Packet and East
    Riding Times*, 21 June 1844, p. 8.

'Superstition at Hull', *The Stamford Mercury*, 14 June 1844, p. 4.

3   A single look in the mirror

'A case was heard at Brentford …', *Nottinghamshire Guardian*,
    12 December 1896, p. 4.

'A Dangerous Beautifier', *Nottingham Evening Post*, 18 October
    1894, p. 2.

'Arsenic eaters', *The Coventry Evening Telegraph*, 20 July 1894,
    p. 2.

'Arsenic for the Complexion', *The Manchester Courier and
    Lancashire General Advertiser*, 23 December 1882, p. 6.

'Arsenical Soap', *Berrow's Worcester Journal*, 12 December 1896,
p. 9.

'Arsenical Soap', *The Lancet*, Vol. 149, 2 January 1897, p. 52.

'Arsenical Soap Again', *The Sheffield Evening Telegraph*,
24 December 1896, p. 3.

'Arsenical Soap Without Arsenic', *The Evening Telegraph*
(Dundee), 10 May 1897, p. 2.

'Cowardly Assault on a Wife', *The Morning Post* (London),
7 October 1893. p. 2.

'Chats on Hygiene', *Myra's Journal*, 1 March 1895, p. 13.

Chemist and Druggist, Vol. 51, 1897, p. 544.

'Dearest Cora', Personal Advertisements, *The Standard*
(London), 16 June 1896, p. 1.

'One Box of Dr Campbell's Harmless Arsenic Wafers', *The Era*
(London), 1 October 1893, p. 11.

'Our Domestic Circle', *The Manchester Courier and Lancashire
General Advertiser: Weekly Supplement*, 25 August 1894, p. 1.

Ship: *Campania*, Arrival: 10 June 1893, *UK Incoming Passenger
Lists, 1878–1960* [database online], Ancestry.com.

Ship: *Circassia*, Arrival: 18 October 1892. *New York, Passenger
Lists, 1820–1957* [database online], Ancestry.com.

'Some Brides Who Are Old: How New York Ladies Retain
Their Beauty So Late', *The New York Times*, 10 April 1887.

'The Brewer and the Lady', *The Hull Daily Mail*, 20 May
1892, p. 3.

'The Arsenic Craze', *Hearth and Home*, 14 January 1897,
p. 396.

---

4   Every affection incidental to the human frame

'A Modest Quack', *The Leicester Chronicle*, 4 September 1841,
p. 4.

A popular Song throughout the Principality of Wales, to
the Baron Spolasco, M.D., A.B., &c. (London), 1840.
Patent Medicines 21 (47). The John Johnson Collection
of Printed Ephemera. Bodleian Library, Oxford. *The John
Johnson Collection: An Archive of Printed Ephemera*. ProQuest.
British Library. 10 November 2012 http://0-johnjohnson.
chadwyck.co.uk.catalogue.wellcomelibrary.org

'Assize Intelligence', *The Hereford Journal*, 29 July 1840, p. 2.

'Baron Spolasco commemorated the anniversary …' *Freeman's
Journal* (Dublin), 1 February 1839, p. 3.

'Dr. Spolasco', Advertisement, *The New York Daily Tribune*,
6 December 1850, p. 1.

John William Adolphus Frederick Augustus Smith, Probate:
1862, *England & Wales, National Probate Calendar (Index of
Wills and Administrations), 1858–1966* [database online],
Ancestry.com.

John William Spolasco, Trial: Glamorgan, 2 March 1839,
England & Wales, Criminal Registers, 1791–1892 [database
online], Ancestry.com.

John William Spolasco, Trial: Glamorgan, 16 July 1840,
England & Wales, Criminal Registers, 1791–1892 [database
online], Ancestry.com.

John Spolasco, London Metropolitan Archives, Lambeth St
Mary, Register of Baptism, p85/mry1, Item 384. *London,
England, Births and Baptisms, 1813–1906* [database online],
Ancestry.com.

'Manslaughter by a Quack, at Bridgend', *The Lancet*, Vol. 31,
23 February 1839, pp. 822–823.

'Police Intelligence of Saturday: Southwark', *The Standard*
(London), 11 June 1849, p. 4.

Ship: *Wisconsin*, Arrival: 2 January 1850, *New York, Passenger
Lists, 1820–1957* [database online], Ancestry.com.

Spolasco, Baron, 'Most Important to all Classes!', Handbill (London), 1848, Patent Medicines 21 (49). The John Johnson Collection of Printed Ephemera Bodleian Library, Oxford, *The John Johnson Collection: An Archive of Printed Ephemera*, ProQuest, British Library, 10 November 2012 http://0-johnjohnson.chadwyck.co.uk.catalogue. wellcomelibrary.org.

Spolasco, Baron, *Narrative of the Wreck of the Steamer Killarney*, F. Jackson, Cork, 2nd edition, 1838.

'Spolasco in Blaenafon', *The Hereford Times*, 26 October 1844, p. 3.

'Spolasco in Custody', *The World (Evening Edition)*, New York, 18 September 1900, p. 1.

Swansea – The Baron Spolasco', *The Era* (London), 15 December 1839, p. 2.

'The celebrated Baron Spolasco was liberated from Cardiff Gaol …', *The Hereford Journal*, 6 March 1839, p. 4.

'The Baron and an Olive Branch', *The Worcestershire Chronicle*, 9 February 1848, p. 5.

'The Last of the (Quack) Barons', *The Cork Examiner*, 5 November 1858, p. 4.

Whitman, Walt, *New York Dissected, A Sheaf of Recently Discovered Newspaper Articles by the Author of Leaves of Grass*, Rufus, Rockwell, Wilson, New York, 1936.

'Wreck of the Killarney – Inquest', *The Bath Chronicle and Weekly Gazette*, 8 February 1838, p. 2.

'Wreck of the Killarney Steamer', *The Morning Post* (London), 6 February 1838, p. 4.

---

5 New life and manly vigour

Acton, William, *The functions and disorders of the reproductive organs in childhood, youth, adult age, and advanced life: considered* in their physiological, social, and moral relations, J. Churchill, London, 3rd edition, 1862.

'An Advertising Surgeon', *The Manchester Times*, 25 September 1869, p. 5.

'A "Secret Friend" Victim', *British Medical Journal*, Vol. 2, No. 200 (29 October 1864), pp. 493–494.

'A "Silent Friend" Silenced', *British Medical Journal*, Vol. 2, No. 205 (3 December 1864), pp. 632–634.

'Copaiba, Cubebs and Capsules entirely superseded. WRAY'S BALSAMIC PILLS', *The Salopian Journal*, 25 February 1862, p. 2.

Courtenay, F. B., *Revelations of Quacks and Quackery: a series of letters by 'Detector'*, Ballière, Tindall and Cox, London, 7th edition, 1877.

'Dr Henery and Co.', *British Medical Journal*, Vol. 2, No. 205 (3 December 1864), p. 641.

'Extraordinary Charge of Extortion', *Reynolds's Newspaper*, 30 October 1864, p. 8.

'Illegal Medical Pretensions', *Reynolds's Newspaper*, 5 October 1879, p. 6.

'London Therapeutic Institution for the Recovery of Health', *The Westmorland Gazette and Kendal Advertiser*, 11 June 1853, p. 7.

Notice under the Bankruptcy Act, 1861, and the Bankruptcy Amendment Act, 1868, *The London Gazette*, 10 August 1869, p. 4468.

Old Bailey Proceedings Online (www.oldbaileyonline.org, version 7.0, 23 January 2013), November 1864, trial of JOHN OSTERFIELD WRAY (28) WILLIAM ANDERSON (42) (t18641121–52).

Old Bailey Proceedings Online (www.oldbaileyonline.org, version 7.0, 23 January 2013), November 1864, trial of JOHN OSTERFIELD WRAY (28) WILLIAM ANDERSON (42) (t18641121–53).

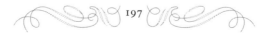

'Phosphorus is the Active Element of Life', *The Norfolk Chronicle*, 25 July 1868, p. 7.

'Police Intelligence: Marlborough Street', *The Morning Post* (London), 22 December 1876, p. 3.

'Suicide from the Perusal of Quack Pamphlets', *The Sheffield Daily Telegraph*, 23 January 1865, p. 4.

'To the British Public. Read This,' *Tamworth Herald*, 27 November 1886, p. 3.

'The Charge of Conspiring to Defraud a Captain', *The Standard* (London), 27 October 1864, p. 7.

'Vital Hints on Health and Strength', by Dr Henery. Pamphlet. (London), 1860–64. Patent Medicines 15 (41). The John Johnson Collection of Printed Ephemera. Bodleian Library, Oxford. *The John Johnson Collection: An Archive of Printed Ephemera*. ProQuest. British Library. 20 Jan. 2013 http://0-johnjohnson.chadwyck.co.uk. catalogue.wellcomelibrary.org.

6   He who can humbug best is the cleverest man

'Annals of Quackery: Cameron, the Water-Taster', *The Medical Adviser, and Guide to Health and Long Life*, No. 4, 27 December 1823, pp. 61–63.

'Annals of Quackery: Report of the Dinner of the New College', *The Medical Adviser, and Guide to Health and Long Life*, No. 51, 13 November 1824, pp. 348–350.

Crell, A.F. & Wallace, W.M., *The Family Oracle of Health: Economy, Medicine, and Good Living*, J. Walker, London, 6th edn, 1824.

Forbes, Duncan, M.D., 'On the Origin and Progress of Empiricism', *The Medical and Physical Journal*, Vol. 15, January–June 1806, pp. 362–370.

'Inward Complaints', Advertisement, *The Morning Chronicle*, 20 September 1819, p. 1.

'It is surprising the number of persons …' Advertisement,
    The Morning Chronicle, 4 April 1815, p. 3.
Jones, James, 'Water-Doctors', *The Monthly Gazette of Health*,
    Vol. 4, No. 47, 1 November 1819, pp. 333–335.
Porter, Roy, *Health for Sale: Quackery in England, 1650–1850*,
    Manchester University Press, Manchester, 1989.

7   To raise false hopes

'Antidipso', *The Lancet*, Vol. 162, 19 December 1903,
    p. 1742.
'Antidipso', *The Lancet*, Vol. 163, 9 January 1904, p. 110.
'"Cures" for Alcoholism', *British Medical Journal*, Vol. 1,
    No. 2249 (6 February 1904), pp. 316–317.
'Drunkenness Cured', Advertisement, *The Penny Illustrated
    Paper*, 17 June 1911, p. 800.
'A Stretcher' *Fun* (London), 17 December 1870, p. 238.
'Great News for Little People', *The Leeds Mercury*,
    10 November 1870, p. 3.
'Mr A.L. Pointing's Will', *Chemist and Druggist*, 13 May 1911,
    p. 632.
'Murray Co., etc.' *Truth*, Vol. 59, 1906, p. 454.
'Occasional Notes', *Pall Mall Gazette*, 16 January 1871, p. 5.
Old Bailey Proceedings Online (www.oldbaileyonline.org,
    version 7.0, 29 September 2012), June 1897, trial of
    ARTHUR LEWIS POINTING (29) (t18970628–461).
'Police Intelligence', *The Morning Post* (London), 10 June
    1874, p. 3.
'Portable Vapour Baths: Burning Accident at Levenshulme',
    The Manchester Evening News, 30 December 1903, p. 2.
Report from the Select Committee on Patent Medicines,
    together with the proceedings of the committee, minutes
    of evidence, and appendices. 1914 (414), IX.1.

'The Composition of Certain Secret Remedies', *British Medical Journal*,Vol. 1, No. 2519, pp. 909–911.

'To Short Persons', Advertisement, *The Daily News* (London), 30 July 1872, p. 4.

---

8   A long life and a busy one

'Barrett's Mandrake Embrocation', Advertisement, *The Leeds Times*, 9 February 1888, p. 8.

'Barrett's Mandrake Embrocation', Handbill (London), 1889. Patent Medicines 1 (33). The John Johnson Collection of Printed Ephemera. Bodleian Library, Oxford. *The John Johnson Collection: An Archive of Printed Ephemera*. ProQuest. British Library. 21 Feb. 2013 http://0-johnjohnson. chadwyck.co.uk.catalogue.wellcomelibrary.org.

'Barrett's Mandrake Embrocation', Handbill (Snaith), 1908. Patent Medicines 1 (34). The John Johnson Collection of Printed Ephemera. Bodleian Library, Oxford. *The John Johnson Collection: An Archive of Printed Ephemera*. ProQuest. British Library. 21 Feb. 2013 http://0-johnjohnson. chadwyck.co.uk.catalogue.wellcomelibrary.org

'Barrett's Pure Mandrake Powder for the Liver', Advertisement, *The Daily Mail* (London), 17 October 1899, p. 8.

Chemist and Druggist,Vol. 36, 1890, p. 621.

'Devon County Show at Torrington', *The Western Times*, 25 May 1895, p. 4.

England Census Records: 1871, 1881, 1891, 1901, and 1911 [database online], Ancestry.com.

Grieve, M., *A Modern Herbal*, Dover Publications, New York, 1971 [first published 1931], published online by Greenwood, E. http://www.botanical.com.

'Influenza, like all troubles which afflict humanity, is loth to leave us …' *The Bristol Mercury*, 14 March 1890, p. 8.

Marriage of Joshua Barrett and Martha Ann Penty, 1919, Fylde, Lancashire, *England & Wales, Marriage Index, 1916–2005* [database online], Ancestry.com.

'Miscellaneous', *Chemist and Druggist*, Vol. 46, 1895, p. 894.

Phelps Brown, O., *The Complete Herbalist, or, The People Their Own Physicians*, Published by the Author, Jersey City, N.J., 1897.

Stables, Gordon, 'The Coming Epidemic or Russian Influenza', *The Reading Mercury*, 4 January 1890.

The Gardener's Chronicle and New Horticulturalist, 14 September 1889, p. 305.

'Wanted, At Once', Advertisement, *The Teesdale Mercury*, 18 September 1918.

---

9   They never came out of the human foot

Ashton, T.J., *A Treatise on Corns, Bunions, and Ingrowing of the Toe-Nail*, John Churchill, London, 1852.

'Attempting to Defraud Mr J W Plunkett', *The Western Daily Press*, 8 January 1877, p. 4.

'Chiropody', *The Lancet*, Vol. 49, Issue 1224, 13 February 1847, pp. 188–189.

'Chiropody Extraordinary, *The Lancet*, Vol. 48, Issue 1217, 26 December 1846, pp. 701–702.

'Curious Charge of Imposture', *The Morning Post* (London), 18 October 1841, p. 4.

Durlacher, Lewis, *A Treatise on Corns, Bunions, the Diseases of the Nails, and the General Management of the Feet*, Simpkin, Marshall and Co., London, 1845.

'From H.R.H. Prince Louis Napoleon', Advertisement, *The Morning Post* (London), 21 May 1849, p. 7.

'Scandalous Imposition', *The Worcester Journal*, 21 October 1841, p. 4.

'Substitute for Corns', *The Lancet*, Vol. 49, Issue 1219, 9 January 1847, p. 51.

'Suffolk Christmas Sessions: The Chiropodist', *The Ipswich Journal*, 9 January 1847, p. 4.

'Trial of Wolff, "The Chiropodist"', *The Essex Standard*, 15 January 1847, p. 4.

'Tricks of Chiropodists', *The Lancet*, Vol. 49, Issue 1219, 9 January 1847, pp. 47–48.

Wake, Robert, 'To the Editor of the *Medical Times*', *The Medical Times*, 20 February 1847, p. 412.

10 Dodging about all over England

'A Little Mistake', *The Hereford Times*, 13 October 1860, p. 9.

'For the Good of Suffering Humanity', *The Illustrated Police News*, 1 June 1872, p. 4.

'More Extraordinary Cases of Taenia or Tapeworm by Baron McKinsey's Botanical Medicines', *The Western Times*, 7 February 1852, p. 2.

'Only that the feat required …', *The Exeter and Plymouth Gazette Daily Telegram*, 3 August 1874, p. 2.

Philp, Robert Kemp, *The Interview: A Companion Volume to 'Enquire Within'*, Houlston and Stoneman, London, 1856.

'Raid upon Obscene Books', *The Exeter and Plymouth Gazette Daily Telegram*, 1 August 1874, pp. 2–3.

'The Cure Effected or Nothing Charged', *The Exeter and Plymouth Gazette*, 15 February 1845, p. 1.

'The Charge Against "Baron" McKinsey', *Trewman's Exeter Flying Post*, 30 April 1884, p. 8.

'Welcome News From America', Advertisement, *The North Devon Journal*, 29 August 1872, p. 7.

11 A source of considerable trouble

'A Bogus Lady Doctor in Birmingham', *The Manchester Courier and Lancashire General Advertiser*, p. 8.

'Alleged Fraud by a "Lady Doctor"', *The Birmingham Daily Post*, 12 April 1892, p. 7.

'Alleged Robbery by a "Lady Doctor"', *Berrow's Worcester Journal*, 16 April 1892, p. 6.

'Attempted Suicide', *The Worcestershire Chronicle*, 20 August 1887, p. 10.

'Credulity at Neath', *The Western Mail*, 10 May 1895, p. 4.

'Curious Case of False Pretences', *The Worcestershire Chronicle*, 9 June 1888, p. 7.

'Curious Charge of False Pretences', *The Derby Daily Telegraph*, 26 February 1890, p. 4.

England and Wales, Criminal Registers, 1791–1892 [database online], Ancestry.com.

England Census Records: 1861, 1871, 1881, 1891, 1901, 1911 [database online], Ancestry.com.

'Gleanings', *The Birmingham Daily Post*, 2 November 1886, p. 7.

'Herefordshire Quarter Sessions: A Herbalist's Case', *The Birmingham Daily Post*, 3 July 1888, p. 5.

'Hereford Quarter Sessions', *The Worcestershire Chronicle*, 7 July 1888, p. 3.

'Jottings', *Berrow's Worcester Journal*, 2 March 1889, p. 5.

'Singular Charge of Fraud', *The Worcestershire Chronicle*, 16 June 1888, p. 7.

'The Bogus Lady Doctor: A Career of Fraud', *The Birmingham Daily Post*, 19 February 1890, p. 3.

'The Quack Doctress Case', *Berrow's Worcester Journal*,
    26 January 1889, p. 7.
'The Sham Lady Doctor', *The Tamworth Herald*, 22 March
    1890, p. 6.

12 You will become like the dainty girl

'A Ludicrous Scene', Advertisement, *The Leeds Mercury*,
    31 May 1879, p. 12.
'By taking daily 3 Capsuloids, there will be produced enough
    Red Blood to fill your Heart', Advertisement, *The Isle of
    Man Times*, 22 December 1900, p. 5.
'Can Stout Women Wear the Sheath Gown?', Advertisement,
    The Manchester Courier and Lancashire General Advertiser,
    12 June 1908, p. 11.
'Dr Campbell's Red Blood Forming Capsuloids',
    Advertisement, *The Gloucester Citizen*, 22 January 1897, p. 3.
'Chancery Division. In re the application of the Capsuloid
    Company (Limited) for registration of a trade mark
    "Tablones, they remove the cause" and in re the Patents,
    Designs and Trade Marks Acts', *The Times*, 30 October
    1906, p. 3.
'Figuroids Cure Obesity', Advertisement, *The Manchester
    Courier and Lancashire General Advertiser*, 9 January 1908,
    p. 9.
'Figuroids', Leaflet [London], *c.* 1907. Patent Medicines 3
    (11). The John Johnson Collection of Printed Ephemera.
    Bodleian Library, Oxford. *The John Johnson Collection: An
    Archive of Printed Ephemera*. ProQuest. British Library.
    23 November 2012 http://0-johnjohnson.chadwyck.
    co.uk.catalogue.wellcomelibrary.org.
'Is Fatness a Social Offence?', Advertisement, *The Daily Mail*
    (London), 6 October 1908, p. 9.

'King's Bench Division: Hansen vs. Dixon', *The Times*, 3 1906, p. 3.

'King's Bench Division: Hansen vs. Dixon', *The Times*, 6 November 1906, p. 14.

'The Composition of Certain Secret Remedies: Obesity Cures', *British Medical Journal*, Vol. 2, No. 2499, 21 November 1908, pp. 1566–1569.

---

13 When exhausted he will bear it in mind

'Ammoniaphone Exhibition', Advertisement, *The Morning Post* (London), 2 July 1885., p. 1.

'"Bottled Italian Air"', *Pall Mall Gazette*, 10 November 1884, p. 5.

'Chemicals and Song: The Marvels of the Ammoniaphone', *Pall Mall Gazette*, 28 July 1884, pp. 11–12.

'Colonel Mapleson's Concert', *The Era* (London), 20 June 1885, p. 9.

'Dr Carter Moffat's Ammoniaphone', Advertisement, *The Dundee Courier*, 23 July 1885, p. 4.

'Dr Carter Moffat's Ammoniaphone', Advertisement, *The Sheffield Daily Telegraph*, 31 July 1885, p. 2.

'In the matter of the Companies Act 1862 to 1890, and in the matter of the Medical Electrical Institute Limited, *The London Gazette*, 12 March 1895, p. 1487.

'Occasional Notes', *Pall Mall Gazette*, 17 January 1884, p. 4.

'Occasional Notes', *Pall Mall Gazette*, 13 June 1885, p. 3.

'New Music', *The Freeman's Journal*, 15 August 1885, p. 6.

'The Ammoniaphone', *The Freeman's Journal*, 4 September 1885, p. 7.

'The Ammoniaphone', *The North-Eastern Daily Gazette* (Middlesbrough), 12 September 1884, p. 3.

'The Ammoniaphone Company (Limited)', *The Western Mail*,
    4 June 1886, p. 3.

'The Ammoniaphone will cure by inhalation', *The Nottingham
    Evening Post*, 8 October 1886, p. 4.

'The Harness Electropathic Swindle' (Series of articles and
    related correspondence), *Pall Mall Gazette*, 19–28 October
    1893.

'The Medical Battery Case: Mr Harness' Medical
    Knowledge', *The Manchester Evening News*, 4 July 1894,
    p. 3.

'The Most Beneficent Invention the World has Ever Known',
    Advertisement, *The Nottingham Evening Post*, 20 November
    1885, p. 4.

14 Thou Church-yard Pimp

Aminicus, 'To the Editors of the Medical and Physical
    Journal', *The Medical and Physical Journal*, Vol. 17, January
    1807, pp. 173–175.

Anon, *Essay on Quackery, and the Dreadful Consequences
    Arising from Taking Advertised Medicines*, T. Clayton, Hull,
    1805.

Antiquack, 'Death from Ching's Worm Lozenges', *The Medical
    Adviser, and Guide to Health and Long Life*, No. 56,
    18 December 1824, pp. 427–428.

'Art. 24: An Essay on Quackery', *The British Critic*, Vol. 25,
    1805, p. 687.

Clayton, M.J., 'To the Editors of the Medical Observer, *The
    Medical Observer*, pp. 401–407.

'Essay on Quackery, and the Dreadful Consequences etc.',
    Review, *The Anti-Jacobin Review and Magazine*, December
    1805, p. 415.

'From Colonel Riddell, Exmouth, Devonshire, to Messrs. Ching and Butler', Advertisement, *The Kentish Gazette*, 11 December 1804, p. 2.

'From Messrs Smart and Cowslade, Reading, to Mr. Ching', Advertisement, *The Reading Mercury*, 17 March 1800, p. 4.

'From the Honourable and Right Reverend the Lord Bishop of Carlisle', Advertisement, *The Reading Mercury*, 6 January 1800, p. 4.

'Mr. John Ching's Worm Lozenges', *The Medical Observer*, No. 2, 1806, pp. 142–155.

15 Making the patient a perfect fright

'J.K.M.', 'Acts of Advertising Dentists', *The Lancet*, Vol. 32, Issue 815, 13 April 1839, p. 112.

Mouland, Luke, *A Londoner's Diary: The Life and Times of a Victorian Bank Clerk*, http://victorianjournal.co.uk/

Bene, C., 'Remarks on the Extraction of Teeth, *The Lancet*, Vol. 20, Issue 507, 18 May 1833, pp. 236–238.

Forbes, Eric G., 'The Professionalization of Dentistry in the United Kingdom', *Medical History*, Vol. 29 (1985), pp. 169–181.

Gray, John, *Dental Advice, with Some Reasons why the Cause of the Defective State of the Teeth, in the Present Day, When compared with the Last Century, May be attributed to Empiricism*, London, 1836.

Gray, John, *Dental Practice, or, Observations on The Qualifications of the Surgeon-Dentist, etc.*, London, 1837.

Richards, N.D., 'Dentistry in England in the 1840s', *Medical History*, Vol. 12 (2) (1968), pp. 137–152.

'Trowbridge County Court', *The Wells Journal*, 26 June 1852, p. 8.

'Dental Quackery', *The Devizes and Wiltshire Gazette*, 17 June 1852, p. 3.

16 Lying round with basins by their heads

Cable Repairing', *The Feilding Star* (Manawatu–Wanganui, NZ), 6 July 1906, p. 4.

'Captain Neagle, formerly in command of a telegraph steamer …', *The Singapore Free Press and Mercentile Advertiser,*' 23 March 1909, p. 8.

'Death After Sea-Sickness', *The Bath Chronicle and Weekly Gazette*, 26 August 1909, p. 4.

'Death From Sea-Sickness', *The Coventry Evening Telegraph*, 16 August 1902, p. 2.

Fordyce Barker, Benjamin, *On Sea-Sickness*, D. Appleton & Co., New York, 1870.

'Hypnotic Cure for Sea-Sickness', *The Aberdeen Journal*, 26 January 1909, p. 6.

'Les Miserables', Advertisement, *The Manchester Courier and Lancashire General Advertiser*, 24 November 1909, p. 3.

'Mer-syren', *The Straits Times*, 26 July 1905, p. 5.

'Mer-Syren Limited', *The London Gazette*, 16 April 1912, p. 2735.

Meyer, Sir William Stevenson et al., *The Imperial Gazetteer of India, Vol. 8, Berhampore to Bombay*, Clarendon Press, Oxford, 1908.

'New Cure for Sea-Sickness', *The Northants Evening Telegraph*, 3 June 1901, p. 4.

'Novel Cure for Sea-Sickness,' *The Edinburgh Evening News*, 3 January 1903, p. 2.

'Say Good-bye to Biliousness, Indigestion and Dyspepsia', Advertisement, *The Manchester Courier and Lancashire General Advertiser*, 16 November 1909, p. 3.

'The Composition of Certain Secret Remedies', *British Medical Journal*, Vol. 1, No. 2631, 3 June 1911, pp. 1324–1325.

'The Cure of Sea-Sickness', *The Northants Evening Telegraph*, 23 February 1901, p. 8.

'The London halfpenny daily is aflame ...' *The Straits Times*, 26 July 1905, p. 1.

'Wonderful 10-Minute Cure', Advertisement, *The Daily Mail* (London), 5 March 1912, p. 7.

17 A place where urine was kept

'Deafness, Noises in Ears', Advertisement, *The Yorkshire Gazette*, 19 December 1857, p. 2.

'Exceedingly imposing was an edifice...', *The Standard* (London), 9 March 1859, p. 4.

'Extraordinary Exposure', *The Reading Mercury*, 12 March 1859, p. 2.

'Police: Hatton Garden', *The Standard* (London), 17 November 1831, p. 4.

The Bennett-Colston-Watters-Skinner-Nicholls-Brandon Gang of Advertising Aurists, *The Medical Times and Gazette*, 19 February 1859, p. 202.

'The Effects of the Bennett Gang', *The Morning Chronicle* (London), 21 March 1859, p. 8.

'The Quackery Villany', *The Lancet*, Vol. 73, Issue 1854, 12 March 1859, pp. 274–275.

Old Bailey Proceedings Online (www.oldbaileyonline. org, version 7.0, 10 October 2012), April 1859, trial of AMBROSE HAYNES, JOHN GIBSON BENNETT, WILLIAM ALFRED BENNETT (t18590404–411).

Old Bailey Proceedings Online (www.oldbaileyonline.org, version 7.0, 10 October 2012), July 1859, trial of JOHN

NICHOL WATTERS (51), CLAUDE EDWARDS (27)
(t18590704–701).

'Scattergood vs. John Gibson Bennett', *The Standard*
(London), 21 February 1859, p. 7.

---

18 To avoid all appearance of puffing

Cartwright, W.A., 'A Case of "Loin Fallen"', *The Veterinarian*,
Vol. 28, No. 325, January 1855, pp. 10–12.

'Cattle, Horses, &c., &c.', Advertisement, *The Hereford Times*,
13 July 1833, p. 1.

'Clarke's Celebrated Herbaceous Liquid', Advertisement,
The Hereford Journal, 16 February 1825, p. 2.

England Census Records: 1841, 1851 [database online],
Ancestry.com.

'I, Francis Macklin…' Advertisement, *The Hereford Journal*,
23 June 1824, p. 3.

'Local News: Deaths', *The Hereford Times*, 10 December 1842,
p. 3.

Marriage of Nathaniel Blaste and Phoebe Clark, 1815,
Warrington, Lancashire, *England & Wales Marriages, 1538–
1940* [database online], Ancestry.com.

Phoebe Blaste, London Metropolitan Archives, Saint
Luke, Old Street, Register of burials, P76/LUK,
Item 074; *London, England, Deaths and Burials, 1813–
1980* [database online], Ancestry.com.

'The "Life's Friend"', Advertisement, *The Hereford Times*,
13 September 1845, p. 1.

19 All came about as I desired

'A Bogus Apothecary', *The Ipswich Journal*, 17 October 1896,
p. 5.

'Advertisements & Notices', *Illustrated Police News*, London,
23 January 1897.

'Alleged Horrible Blackmailing Plot', *Royal Cornwall Gazette
Falmouth Packet, Cornish Weekly News, & General Advertiser*,
Truro, 24 November 1898.

'Alleged Illegal Operation', *Reynolds's Newspaper*,
28 November 1897, p. 7.

'An Edinburgh Licentiate Struck off the Rolls, *The Dundee
Courier*, 11 June 1896, p. 5.

'A Vile Trade', *The Bath Chronicle and Weekly Gazette*,
20 January 1898, p. 5.

Bradlaugh, Charles, and Besant, Annie (eds), *The Queen vs.
Charles Bradlaugh and Annie Besant*, Freethought Publishing
Company, London, 1877.

'Charge of Extorting Money', *The Times*, London,
17 November 1898.

'Doctors Sent to Penal Servitude', *Lloyd's Weekly Newspaper*,
23 January 1898, p. 15.

Knight, Patricia, 'Women and Abortion in Victorian and
Edwardian England', *History Workshop*, No. 4, 1977, 57–68.

Lambert, E.J., *Special List of Domestic and Surgical Specialities*,
Lambert & Son, Dalston, London, *c.* 1891. Patent
Medicines 18 (48). The John Johnson Collection of Printed
Ephemera. Bodleian Library, Oxford. *The John Johnson
Collection: An Archive of Printed Ephemera*. ProQuest. British
Library. 2 August 2012 http://0-johnjohnson.chadwyck.
co.uk.catalogue.wellcomelibrary.org.

Manvell, Roger, *The Trial of Annie Besant and Charles Bradlaugh*,
Elek/Pemberton, London, 1976.

McLaren, Angus, *Birth Control in Nineteenth-Century England*, Croom Helm Ltd, London, 1978.

Porter, Roy, and Hall, Lesley, *The Facts of Life: The Creation of Sexual Knowledge in Britain, 1650–1950*, Yale University Press, New Haven and London, 1995.

'Quacks and Abortion: A Critical and Analytical Enquiry', *The Lancet*, Vol. 152, Issues. 3928, 3929, 3930, 3931; 1898, pp. 1570–71, 1651–53, 1723–24, 1807–08.

'The Magic Female Pills', Advertisement, *The Aberdeen Journal*, 29 October 1890, p. 4.

'"The Worst Newspaper in England"', *Pall Mall Gazette*, London, 23 November 1886.

'Thomasso's Perfect Cure is now Thrilling the Country', Advertisement, *The Aberdeen Journal*, 8 October 1890, p. 1.

'Thomasso's Perfect Cure', Leaflet, 1890, *British Library Evanion Collection of Ephemera*.

'On the route of the Procession. Patent medicine Vendor and his Debts', *The Gloucester Citizen*, 18 June 1897, p. 4.

20 A new man after one vigorous application

'Anti-Stiff', *Chemist and Druggist*, Vol. 36, 1890, p. 711.

'Anti-Stiff', *Fun*, 27 May 1891, p. 217.

Cleopatra, 'Cycling Gossip', *Bow Bells: A Magazine of General Literature and Art for Family Reading*, 13. 164, 20 February 1891, p. 79.

Cleopatra, 'Cycling Gossip', *Bow Bells: A Magazine of General Literature and Art for Family Reading*, 1. 140, 5 September 1890, p. 227.

Cleopatra, 'Cycling Gossip', *Bow Bells: A Magazine of General Literature and Art for Family Reading*, 33. 429, 20 March 1896, p. 309.

Edwardes, Charles, 'The New Football Mania', *The Nineteenth Century: A Monthly Review*, 32. 188, October 1892, pp. 622–631.

'Lady Cyclists', *British Medical Journal*, 7 July 1894, p. 35.

'Lady Cyclists', *The York Herald*, 25 November 1895, p. 6.

'Lady Cyclists and Public-Houses', *The Grantham Journal*, 14 June 1902, p. 2.

'No Athlete can Afford to Ignore Anti-Stiff', The London Pavilion, programme for Monday (amended to Saturday), October 12th (amended to 17th), 1891, London Playbills London Pavilion (6), The John Johnson Collection of Printed Ephemera. Bodleian Library, Oxford. *The John Johnson Collection: An Archive of Printed Ephemera*. ProQuest. British Library. 31 January 2013 http://0-johnjohnson. chadwyck.co.uk.catalogue.wellcomelibrary.org.

'Under the name of "anti-stiff" ...' *The Western Druggist*, Vol. 18, 1896, p. 313.

'Use Anti-Stiff!!', Advertisement, *Cycling*, Vol. 1, No. 1, 24 January 1891, p. 10.

'Who Uses Anti-Stiff? Every Athlete of Note', Advertisement, *The Blackburn Standard*, 2 January 1892, p. 6.

Wanderer, 'Sports and Pastimes', *The Blackburn Standard*, 20 December 1890, p. 6.

21 A horse for every home

'"Mechanical" Horse Exercise', *The Standard* (London), 21 February 1894, p. 2.

'Horse exercise in the home', Advertisement, *The Cornishman*, 12 November 1903, p. 1.

'How to Enjoy Influenza', Advertisement, *Pall Mall Gazette*, 13 March 1895, p. 6.

'It is difficult to believe that any exercise, or pleasure, can in any way equal that of Riding', *Le Follet: Journal du Grande Monde*, 1 May 1895, p. 10.

'There is no exercise so invigorating…' *Hearth and Home*, 29 October 1896, p. 906.

'Town and Country Gossip', *Horse and Hound*, 16 June 1894, p. 369.

Vigor and Co., 'Don't Ride Horses but Ride the Hercules Horse Action Saddle', Leaflet, 1894, *British Library Evanion Collection of Ephemera*.

'Vigor's Home-Rower', Advertisement, *The Graphic* (London), 8 February 1896, p. 183.

22 Their wheels a compilation of human bones

'Advertisers', *The Monthly Gazette of Health*, November 1822, pp. 338–339.

'Annals of Quackery', *The Medical Adviser and Guide to Health and Long Life*, No. 5, 3 January 1824, pp. 78–80.

'A True Blessing to Mankind …', Advertisement, *Woolmer's Exeter and Plymouth Gazette*, 10 November 1832, p. 1.

'Balsam Rakasiri', *The Monthly Gazette of Health*, January 1824, pp. 784–790.

'Base and Malicious Charge of Fraud Refuted', *The Morning Chronicle* (London), 28 February 1829, p. 3.

'Cordial Balm of Rakasiri', *The Medical Adviser and Guide to Health and Long Life*, No. 16, 20 March 1824. p. 250–251.

'"Dr." Jordan', *The Medical Adviser and Guide to Health and Long Life*, No. 19, 10 April 1824, pp. 302–303.

'London College of Health', Advertisement, *The Spectator*, No. 263, 13 July 1833, p. 650.

'Messrs May vs Doctors J and C Jordan, Physicians to the West-London Medical Establishment, and Proprietors of the celebrated Balsam of Rakasiri, &c., &c., &c.,!!!' *The Monthly Gazette of Health*, 1 April 1829, pp. 522–533.

'On Thursday Mr Cox, a solicitor, applied to the Magistrates at Marlborough-street Police Office ...', *The Hampshire Chronicle*, 23 February 1829, p. 4.

'Quackery', *The Examiner* (London), 8 March 1829, p. 13.

'Quackery, &c.', *The Monthly Gazette of Health*, June 1829, pp. 591–592.

'The advertising *Doctors Jordan* ...', *The Examiner* (London), 1 March 1829, p. 14.

'To the Editor of the Morning Chronicle', *The Morning Chronicle*, 5 March 1829, p. 4.

23 Its power to assuage maternal pain

'Alleged Poisoning from an "Infant Preservative"', *British Medical Journal*, 13 March 1886, pp. 511–512.

'Another Victim to Godfrey's Cordial', *The Derbyshire Times and Chesterfield Herald*, 28 June 1878, p. 6.

Atkinson and Barker's Royal Infants Preservative, Handbill, 1872, Food 12 (46). The John Johnson Collection of Printed Ephemera. Bodleian Library, Oxford. The John Johnson Collection: An Archive of Printed Ephemera. ProQuest. British Library. 10 August 2012 http://0-johnjohnson.chadwyck.co.uk.catalogue.wellcomelibrary.org.

'Baby Farming in Manchester', *British Medical Journal*, 22 February 1868, p. 174.

Beasley, Henry, *The Druggist's General Receipt Book*, J.A. Churchill, London, 8th Edition, 1878.

Berridge, Virginia, *Opium and the People: opiate use and drug control policy in nineteenth and early twentieth-century England*, London, Free Association Books, 1999.

Berridge, Virginia, 'Opium Eating and the Working Class in the Nineteenth Century: The Public and Official Reaction', *British Journal of Addiction*, Vol. 73 (1978), pp. 107–112.

Berridge, Virginia, 'Victorian Opium Eating: Responses to Opiate Use in Nineteenth-century England, *Victorian Studies*, Vol. 21 (1978), pp. 437–481.

Chepaitis, Elia Vallone, 'The Opium of the Children: domestic opium and infant drugging in early Victorian England.' Doctoral thesis. University of Connecticut, 1985.

Children's Employment Commission. First report of the commissioners. Mines. 1842 (380) (381) (382) XV.1, XVI.1, XVII.1.

Children's Employment Commission. Second report of the commissioners. Trades and manufactures. 1843 (430) (431) (432) XIII.307, XIV.1, XV.1.

'Day Nursing and Baby Farming', *Lloyd's Weekly Newspaper*, 19 April 1868.

Dr Benjamin Godfrey's Cordial, prepared by Benjamin Godfrey Windus (the sole proprietor), *c.* 1830–1850. Patent Medicines 3 (35). The John Johnson Collection of Printed Ephemera. Bodleian Library, Oxford. *The John Johnson Collection: An Archive of Printed Ephemera*. ProQuest. British Library. 10 August 2012 http://0-johnjohnson.chadwyck. co.uk.catalogue.wellcomelibrary.org.

'Factory Acts Amendment Bill', HC Deb (3rd Series), 11 June 1873, Vol. 216, cc. 819–28.

'Godfrey's Cordial Again', *The Morning Chronicle* (London), 12 September 1856, p. 5.

Halliday, Andrew, 'Mothers', *All the Year Round*, Vol. XIV, 9 September 1865, pp. 157–9.

Hewitt, Margaret, *Wives and Mothers in Victorian Industry* (London, Rockliff, *c.* 1958).

'Hours of Labour in Factories', HC Deb (3rd Series), 15 March 1844, Vol. 73, cc. 1074–1155.

'Infantile Mortality and Summer Diarrhoea', *Leicester Chronicle and the Leicestershire Mercury*, 9 November 1878.

Jerrold, William Blanchard, 'Protected Cradles', *Household Words*, Vol. II (26 October 1850), pp. 108–112.

Lomax, Elizabeth, 'The uses and abuses of opiates in Nineteenth-Century England', *Bulletin of the History of Medicine*, Vol. 47(2) (1973), pp. 167–76.

Mayhew, Henry, 'Labour and the Poor', *The Morning Chronicle*, 15 November 1849.

'Motherhood', *Trewman's Exeter Flying Post or Plymouth and Cornish Advertiser*, 15 February 1865.

Platt, William H., 'A Pernicious System', *British Medical Journal*, 11 March 1876, p. 340.

Public health. Fifth report of the Medical Officer of the Privy Council. With appendix, 1863 (161), XXV.1.

Report from the Select Committee on Protection of Infant Life, 1871 (372), VII.607.

Second report of the commissioners inquiring into the State of Large Towns and Populous Districts. 1845 (602) (610) XVIII.1.

'The Massacre of the Innocents', *Reynolds's Newspaper*, 26 June 1870.

'The Mother's Calling', *The British Mother's Journal*, February 1860, pp. 37–39.

'To The Ladies – The Celebrated Manchester Medicine, Atkinson and Barker's Royal Infants Preservative', Advertisement, *The Coventry Herald*, 6 August 1847, p. 3.

24 The plains are bountiful in bulbs

Ali Ahmed's Treasures of the Desert [London], 1853. Patent
   Medicines 1 (6a). The John Johnson Collection of Printed
   Ephemera. Bodleian Library, Oxford. *The John Johnson
   Collection: An Archive of Printed Ephemera*. ProQuest. British
   Library. 14 December 2012 http://0-johnjohnson.
   chadwyck.co.uk.catalogue.wellcomelibrary.org.
'Ali Ahmed's Treasure of the Desert', Advertisement, *The Leeds
   Intelligencer*, 16 October 1853, p. 3.
Cooley, Arnold J., and Brough, J.C., *Cooley's Cyclopaedia of
   Practical Receipts, Processes, and Collateral Information in the
   Arts, Manufactures, Professions and Trades, including Medicine,
   Pharmacy and Domestic Economy*, John Churchill and Sons,
   London, 4th Edition, 1864.
Darwin, Bernard, *The Dickens Advertiser: A Collection of the
   Advertisements in the Original Parts of Novels by Charles
   Dickens*, Macmillan, New York, 1930.
Neale, Frederick Arthur, *Narrative of a Residence in Siam*, Office
   of the National Illustrated Library, London, 1852.
'Thousands of Cures are Effected by the Use of Ali Ahmed's
   Treasures', Advertisement, *The Bucks Herald*, 18 March
   1854, p. 4.

25 No one could suppose he meant any harm

'Cancer, etc.', Advertisement, *The Elgin Courier*, 8 September
   1865, p. 4.
'Culpable Homicide by a Quack Doctor', *The Glasgow Herald*,
   26 September 1868, p. 4.
'Death of a Cancer Doctor', *The Aberdeen Journal*, 26 August
   1874, p. 6.

'Death from the use of Arsenic by a Cancer Quack', *The Medical News and Library*, Vol. 26, No. 311, November 1868, p. 159.

Gosse, Philip Henry, *A Memorial of the Last Days on Earth of Emily Gosse. By Her Husband,* J Nisbet & Co., London, 1857.

Graham, Thomas, M.D., 'Case of Poisoning by Arsenic, externally applied', *The Glasgow Medical Journal*, Vol. 1, 1869, pp. 56–59.

'Mr Paterson, Cancer Doctor', Advertisement, *The Belfast News-letter*, 7 June 1873, p. 2.

'Mr Paterson, of the Cancer Institution', Advertisement, *The Dundee Advertiser*, 19 October 1866.

'Report of the Middlesex Hospital on Cancer, as treated by Dr Fell', *The Era*, 6 December 1857, p. 10.

'The Black Doctor', *The Morning Post* (London), 7 January 1860, p. 7.

'The Black Doctor Condemned', *The Wells Journal*, 9 April 1859, p. 3.

Wells, Thomas Spencer, *Cancer Cures and Cancer Curers*, London, 1860.

INDEX

INDEX

If you enjoyed this book, you may also be interested in …

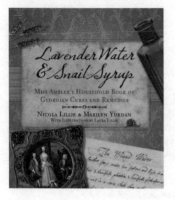

Lavender Water & Snail Syrup

Elizabeth Ambler started compiling her
household book of cures in the early eighteenth
century, including in it treatments which were
much older and had been passed down to her.
These intriguing remedies include Sir Walter
Raleigh's Receipt against Plague, Viper Broth,
Snail Milk Water and Tobacco for the Eyes.
In addition to traditional flowers and herbs,
ingredients consist of precious stones, exotic
and expensive spices, and large amounts of
brandy and wine. Mrs Ambler's book of cures
is exceptional in that has been handed down
through her female descendants over nearly
three centuries.

978 0 7524 8995 7

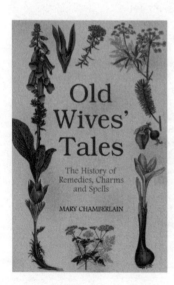

Old Wives' Tales

The woman healer is as old as history. For
millennia she has been doctor, nurse and
midwife, and even in the age of modern
medicine her wisdom is handed down in the
form of old wives' tales. Using extensive research
into archives and original texts, and numerous
conversations with women, Mary Chamberlain
presents a stimulating challenge to the history of
orthodox medicine and an illuminating survey
of female wisdom which goes back to the
earliest times. What are old wives' tales? Where
do they come from? Do they really work? These
questions, and many more, are answered in this
fascinating compendium of remedies and cures
handed down from mother to daughter from the
beginning of time.

978 0 7524 5809 0

Visit our website and discover thousands of
other History Press books.

www.thehistorypress.co.uk

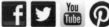